Talking About
Health and Wellness
with Patients

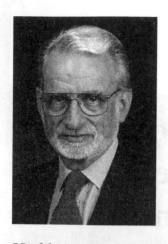

Steven Jonas, MD, MPH, is Professor of Preventive Medicine, School of Medicine, State University of New York at Stony Brook, where he has been a faculty member since 1971. Born and raised in New York City, he received his B.A. from Columbia College in 1958, his M.D. from the Harvard Medical School in 1962, his M.P.H. from the Yale School of Medicine in 1967, and his M.S. in Health Management from New York University in 1997.

He is Fellow of the American College of Preventive Medicine, the American Public Health Association, and the New York Academy of Medicine. He is Editor of the Springer *Series on Medical Education*, an Associate Editor of *Preventive Medicine*, a member of the editorial board and a regular columnist for the *American Athletics Association Quarterly*, and a member of the Editorial Board of *ACSM's Health and Fitness Journal*. He is a Past President of the Association of Teachers of Preventive Medicine and a past member of the New York State Board for Medicine.

Dr. Jonas is Founding Editor of *Jonas-Kovner: Health Care Delivery in the United States* (published by Springer Publishing), was Editor and Coauthor of its first three editions, and is Coeditor of the Sixth Edition (1998) and the Seventh Edition (forthcoming in 2002). He has authored nine books of his own, including *Medical Mystery: The Training of Doctors in the United States* (1978), *Regular Exercise: A Handbook for Clinical Practice* (published by Springer Publishing, 1995), *The Essential Triathlete* (1996), and *An Introduction to the U.S. Health Care System*, Fourth Edition (published by Springer Publishing, 1998). He is author or coauthor of ten books on health promotion, exercise, and weight management.

On health policy, preventive medicine, and drug abuse policy, Dr. Jonas has published over 100 professional articles and book reviews and delivered over 75 papers at conferences and seminars. He has also published numerous articles and given many talks on sports, exercise promotion, and weight management. He was a designated speaker on behalf of the National Health Care Campaign for the Clinton Health Plan in 1994.

Talking About Health and Wellness with Patients

Integrating Health Promotion and Disease Prevention into Your Practice

Steven Jonas, MD, MPH

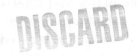

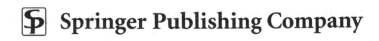

Springer Publishing Company

Springer Publishing Company, Inc.
536 Broadway
New York, NY 10012-3955

Acquisitions Editor: Bill Tucker
Production Editor: Helen Song
Cover design by James Scotto-Lavino

00 01 02 03 04 / 5 4 3 2 1

Library of Congress Cataloging-in-Publication Data

Jonas, Steven.
    Talking about health and wellness with patients: integrating health promotion and disease prevention into your practice / Steven Jonas.
        p.   cm.
    Includes bibliographical references and index.
    ISBN 0-8261-1338-9 (softcover)
    1. Health promotion.   2. Medicine, Preventive.
3. Clinical health psychology.   4. Health.   I. Title.

RA427.8 .J66 2000
613—dc21
                                        99-087585

Printed in the United States of America

*For Chezna—who has brought the full measure
of health and wellness to my life.*

CONTENTS

FOREWORD

Physicians and other health professionals increasingly encounter opportunities to assist patients and clients in achieving health and wellness. Incorporating into their practices the concepts that Steven Jonas advances in this book will help clinicians take advantage of such opportunities.

In fact they are not merely clinical opportunities; more and more of those who seek professional help for health insist upon obtaining guidance in attaining health and wellness themselves, that is, in addition to overcoming disease. The reason for this tendency is the changing nature of the health problem in America and other industrialized countries. Many people, having escaped death from the diseases that killed their grandparents (tuberculosis, typhoid, and the like) and even their parents (heart disease, cancer, and stroke) now live typically until their late 70's; increasing numbers live into their 80's and 90's with good health. Heart disease, cancer and stroke, of course, are still major causes of death, but mortality from them is now sharply declining.

Beginning to appreciate this new situation, people want more from their health professionals than just overcoming or even avoiding disease. They desire buoyant good health; energy to do the things they like; living on the positive side, not just evading the negative. They emulate those with zest for life of whom they see more and more around them. This is no fad; it is a response to demographic reality.

Unfortunately the vast majority of health professionals now practicing need substantial reorientation to a situation for which they received inadequate training. Their education focused on the complaint-response circumstance: The patient comes with some complaint such as symptom or sign, with need for response in the form of diagnosis and treatment. Even though that type of circumstance still occupies the majority of health professionals' time, people are pursuing more and deserve more.

Fortunately we all know a good deal about what personal behaviors largely determine health and wellness, or the opposite. The problem for many health professionals, however, lies in not knowing how to help their individual patients and clients effectively achieve healthful behavior and a wellness lifestyle. A practical approach toward raising the level of competence in that regard among health professionals is therefore much needed, and is the aim of this book. Indeed, this book's approach to being well and becoming healthy should be of interest and use not only to health professional practitioners and students, but to the sophisticated lay reader as well. This guide to personal health-promoting behavior change will substantially augment the social endeavors now underway to improve the milieu in which people make decisions about tobacco use, exercise, nutrition, alcohol use, and the like. Both one-on-one and broad, social efforts are necessary to make health and wellness widely achievable.

Lester Breslow, MD, MPH
Dean Emeritus and Professor
UCLA School of Public Health

PREFACE

This short book is about personal health promotion/disease prevention (HP/DP) in clinical practice. It is addressed to a broad range of students and clinicians in the health care professions, including: medicine, nursing, physician assisting, social work, psychotherapy, physical therapy, occupational therapy, dentistry, chiropractic, homeopathy, and naturopathy.

To a greater or lesser extent, each member of these professions has the opportunity to address HP/DP in the course of their practices with patients/clients (and many do so). But while in most health professional education programs the nature of disease is well-covered, the nature of health, wellness, and HP/DP is often neglected to a greater or lesser extent. Intended to help remedy this deficiency, this book can be used both as an introductory student textbook and as a guide for practicing clinicians who want to learn about the field, introduce HP/DP into their practice, or, if they have already done so, perhaps improve their work.

For individual patients and clients the primary focus of personal health promotion/disease prevention is changing one or more health-related behaviors. The clinician's key to helping people do this is effective communication. To be an effective communicator, the clinician obviously first must have good communication skills, from speaking clearly to presenting information in a nonthreatening, cooperative, encouraging, change-facilitating manner.

The first major premise of this book is that good communication skills, while necessary, are not sufficient. The clinician must also have a thorough understanding of the nature of the subject about which she or he is communicating, in this case health, wellness, and HP/DP, and how people go about making change in their health-related personal behaviors. Often, guides for clinicians in HP/DP focus almost exclusively on the latter.

The second major premise of this book is that to best help patients and clients to make positive changes in their lives, an understanding of the simple behavioral approaches to behavior change, while necessary, is by itself also not enough. It is postulated that a thorough understanding of the theoretical basis of the field, of both its substance and its processes (which happen to subsume the behavioral approach), and how to apply that understanding in practice, will enable the clinician to better help his or her patients and clients deal with the subject at hand.

This is thought to be so, regardless of which specific behavior-change intervention a clinician might be engaged in, be it, for example, smoking cessation, weight management, or exercise promotion. It is to meeting the need for a clear understanding of this theoretical material, and helping the clinician to use this understanding to effectively communicate with patients and clients, that this book is addressed.

The third major premise of this book is that the theoretical basis of health, wellness, and health promotion/disease prevention can be set forth in capsule form, in what I call the "Ten Central Concepts of Health Promotion/Disease Prevention." Seven describe its elemental substance, three its basic processes. These "Ten Concepts" form the basis of the book's whole argument.

The fourth major premise of this book is a well known reality: There is a single common mental pathway underlying most personal behavior change efforts. It is often referred to as "The Stages of Change," the name given to it by its original describers/discoverers, Drs. J.O. Prochaska and C.C. DiClemente. This pathway is summarized in Concepts VIII, IX, and X, and its application is elucidated in some detail in the book.

The thinking that I share with you here is the product of work that I have been doing off and on over the past 25 years or so. I welcome each reader to the book and hope you will find it useful in the course of your studies and work.

Steven Jonas, MD, MPH, MS
Stony Brook, NY
December 14, 1999

NOTES

The term "patients" and "clients" are used interchangeably in the text. As stated at the beginning of the Preface, this book is addressed to that very broad range of health professions and professionals that engage in HP/DP-related clinical practice. Some refer to the people for whom they provide care as "patients." Others use the term "clients." And so in this book both are used.

Chapters two and three of this book are based in part on adaptations of previously published work of mine, found in chapter two of *Medical Mystery: The Training of Doctors in the United States* (S. Jonas, New York: WW Norton, 1978) and in chapter two of *Jonas' Health Care Delivery in the United States* (5th ed.; A.R. Kovner (Ed.), New York: Springer Publishing Co., 1995).

ACKNOWLEDGMENTS

I wish to thank the following people for their contributions to and encouragement of this endeavor: My long-time publisher and loyal friend, Dr. Ursula Springer, my editors at Springer, Bill Tucker and Helen Song, my friends and colleagues John Hanc and Linda Konner, and my fellow staff members at Stony Brook, Marcia Wiener, Peter Mastroianni, Tejus Sonawala, and all of the other members of the Campus-Wide Wellness Program Planning Committee of the State University of New York, an entity that I have had the privilege to chair.

INTRODUCTION AND DEFINITIONS

Chapter 1

INTRODUCTION

I. WHAT'S IT ALL ABOUT?

Health and wellness. You know the drill. If one does them right the risk of contracting a wide variety of diseases can be reduced, or at least their onset can be delayed. Various aspects of healthy living can improve one's fitness level, help in weight loss, improve physical appearance, enable the handling of life's stresses more productively, lead to a better family life, and so on and so forth. Finally, perhaps the most important benefit of healthy living is that most who do it feel better and feel better about themselves, now.

In 1996, referring to regular exercise, the Surgeon General of the United States, Dr. Audrey Manley (United States Department of Health and Human Service, 1996) put it this way:

> Scientists and doctors have known for years that substantial benefits can be gained from regular physical activity. . . . We have today strong evidence to indicate that regular physical activity will provide clear and substantial health gains. (p. v)

To say nothing of the "feel good" gains.

Yet while most Americans know that what Dr. Manley said is true, not only in terms of physical activity, but also in terms of the wide range of health promoting behaviors, not too many Americans act on the available knowledge. Thus not too many of us lead a balanced, healthy lifestyle. However, that Americans as a people are not particularly healthy in terms of risk-factor control, for example, is not due to a lack of effort in providing information about health and wellness to them. Many, many books and articles on both subjects have been written, are being written, and will be written, to say nothing of all the information that appears every day on TV, on radio, in the newspapers, and on the Internet.

There are in fact a host of reasons why Americans are not a particularly healthy population when it comes to such matters as body weight, diet, physical activity, stress-handling capability, and alcohol abuse, for example. Many personal, societal, and environmental factors are on the list. But among the reasons also is the approach of many in the health professions who, if they deal with the subject at all, often focus on the strictly behavioral method: "Just follow this series of practical steps in eating, or exercise, or stress management, and you will arrive at the desired endpoint."

The instructions (and they are often just that, *instructions*) concern almost entirely *what* to do, with little attention paid to either understanding what health and wellness are or the mental processes required in order to engage in them. This book is constructed on a different premise: that an understanding of both the nature of healthy living and the mental process underlying successful personal behavior change is for many people essential if they are going to get where they want to go. This book is designed to help health professionals and health professions students acquire that central understanding themselves, and in turn to equip them to help their patients/clients acquire it as well.

II. WHAT THIS BOOK IS ABOUT

This book is about personal health and wellness, about the mental processes underlying personal behavior change, and about how clinicians can productively talk about these subjects with patients and clients. At any given time, the health status of an individual is determined by three broad groups of factors: genetic, environmental, and personal/behavioral. All are important. All are constantly interacting with each other over time in a complex, dynamic, three-dimensional feed-back loop.

Health (or lack of it) is, of course, a characteristic not just of individuals but also of groups of people. Thus the health status of communities, societies, nations, geographic regions, and the Earth itself, as well as that of individuals, can be analyzed and described. And the health status of each level of social organization has an impact on the health of each member of the human species, to a greater or lesser extent depending on where one lives and what one's socioeconomic status is.

This book, however, does not take on health globally. Rather, it focuses on personal health, with the major emphasis being on what a person can do to promote his or her own health. At the same time, both the genetic and environmental factors influencing personal health will be discussed as relevant and necessary.

As Dr. Lester Breslow (1996) has said:

> [L]ifestyle consists of ways of living, the patterns of behavior, in the circumstances of one's life. Increasingly in industrialized society we create for ourselves, individually and collectively, both the circumstances of life and our ways of living in those circumstances. And we are beginning to recognize that both those facets of lifestyle strongly influence how long we live and how well.

Within the realm of personal health, recognizing full well that they do not comprise the whole story, the book's primary focus is on that group of health-influencing behavioral factors that are or can be under a person's control. We will examine how they affect one's health, how people can make changes in their own behavior(s) to promote their own health, and how clinical practitioners of all kinds can help them to do that.

The straightforward cognitive/behavioral approach to individual behavior and behavior change (Blair, 1991; Ferguson, 1988; Halper, 1980; Liebman, 1999; Simmons, 1999) has much popularity in the United States. It has much to recommend it, too, at least for certain patients/clients. This book takes a somewhat different approach, however, as noted at the outset of this chapter. That approach is based on the assumption that going beyond the purely behavioral approach will significantly strengthen the hand of the health professional in facilitating positive change in personal health-related behaviors.

The premise is that if, before engaging in straight behavioral interventions, the clinician first has a solid understanding of the theoretical basis of the subject at hand he or she will be better equipped to help the patient/client to improve their health. Further, it is postulated that the same understanding, shared with patients and clients by the knowledgeable health professional, can help many of them in their own behavior change endeavors. Hopefully, the "Ten Central Concepts of Health Promotion/Disease Prevention" presented and elaborated on in this book will provide for the reader a framework for the development of that theoretical understanding in both the substantive and process sectors of the health and wellness arena.

There is nothing magical or mystical about these Ten Concepts. For the most part, each one simply restates an element of received wisdom about the substance and processes of health and wellness and how people can become healthy and well. The central ideas here are that theory can inform practice and be the handmaiden of it, and that the active use of theory on a day-to-day basis can make practice both better for the patient/client and more rewarding, fun if you will, for the practitioner.

III. THE ORGANIZATION OF THE BOOK

Aiming to achieve these goals, this book has three sections. The first comprises chapters 1, 2, and 3. After this chapter, which offers a brief overview of the book, chapter 2 explores some of the definitions of health and wellness that have been offered over time, and of several related terms/concepts, such as disease and illness. Then, in chapter 3, we consider the question "Why Health Promotion/Disease Prevention?"

These chapters are devoted entirely to definitions and some history and policy analysis. Readers interested in these subjects should find them to be of use. However, the material in them that is essential to clinical practice is incorporated into sections two and three of the book. Thus those readers for whom considering alternative definitions of terms and the historic approach is not high on the to-do list can skip chapters 2 and 3 entirely. They would then proceed directly to the applications portion of the book that begins with chapter 4. Such readers could consider coming back to the detailed definitional material later, if the applications sections have piqued their interest in it.

The second section of the book, chapters 4 and 5, is devoted to explaining and analyzing the theoretic basis of the personal health promotion/disease prevention (HP/DP) interventions as they can be applied to help individuals achieve health and wellness. As stated above, this material is formulated as the "Ten Central Concepts of Health Promotion/Disease Prevention."

The third section, comprising chapters 6 through 8, shows how the Ten Central Concepts can be applied in practice to help patients/clients take control of their lives and make personal health promoting behavior change(s). The discussion of using the Ten Central Concepts in effectively communicating with patients/clients about personal HP/DP begins with a presentation (chapter 6) of the primary functions of the health professional during the encounter with an individual client/patient.

Next, chapter 7 illustrates how, in this case using as the example helping a patient or client to become a regular exerciser, the Ten Concepts themselves can be applied in a given clinical situation. The book concludes, in chapter 8, with a consideration of the process the health professional should/could go through if he or she is to routinely include health promotive/disease preventive interventions in personal practice.

IV. THE TEN CENTRAL CONCEPTS OF HEALTH PROMOTION/DISEASE PREVENTION

Just so you, dear reader, will not be on tenterhooks wondering just what the Ten Concepts are, finally in this chapter, I will present them here before proceeding to the main body of the text. Also, later in the book, Concepts I–VII are presented in some detail in chapter 4, VIII–X in chapter 5. And so the Ten Central Concepts of Health Promotion/Disease Prevention:

I. Health is a state of being; wellness is a process of being.
II. Health status is determined by a broad range of factors.
III. Health has a natural history.
IV. Central to the wellness process is a wide array of interventions.
V. Success in certain behavior change endeavors is relative.
VI. Risks to health can be reduced; in few instances is there certainty of outcome.
VII. Achieving balance is the essence of healthy living and wellness.
VIII. There is a common pathway to success for most personal behavior change efforts.
IX. Motivation is a process, not a thing.
X. Assessment, goal setting, and mobilizing motivation are the central tasks in personal behavior change.

The Ten Central Concepts fall into two groups. The first seven are the primarily "substantive" common denominators of healthy and well living. These concepts define and describe what health and wellness *are* and are about, what their theoretic and philosophic *substance* is, and how they (that is, health and wellness) may be characterized and understood, both in individuals and in the abstract. The *process* concepts are the common denominators of how individuals go about changing their personal health-related behaviors. They describe the mental route one takes to get to a healthy/well state of being, using the seven substantive concepts to inform the process. These last three concepts thus deal with just how one goes about becoming and being both healthy and well, about how to incorporate health and wellness into one's life, on the personal level.

Of course, each concept has elements of both substance and process, but they are grouped according to which element is the most prominent in each concept. To lay the groundwork for understanding the Ten Central Concepts and how to use them, I will now turn to the definitions of the term *health* and its relatives that have been developed by a number of authorities over time.

REFERENCES

Blair, S. N. (1991). *Living With exercise*. Dallas, TX: American Health Publishing Co.

Breslow, L. (1996). Social ecological strategies for promoting healthy lifestyles. *American Journal of Health Promotion, 10,* 253.

Ferguson, J. M. (1988). *Habits not diets: The secret to lifetime weight control*. Palo Alto, CA: Bull.

Halper, M. S. (1980). *How to stop smoking*. New York: Holt, Rinehart, and Winston.

Liebman, B. (1999, July/August). Ten tips for staying lean. *Nutrition Action Health Letter, 26,* 1.

Simmons, R. (1999, July). Burn fat faster. *Richard Simmons and Friends, 5,* 8.

U.S. Department of Health and Human Services. (1996). *Physical activity and health*. Atlanta, GA: Centers for Disease Control and Prevention.

Chapter 2

WHAT ARE HEALTH AND WELLNESS?

I. DEFINITIONS OF HEALTH

In this chapter I lay the groundwork for the understanding of the Ten Central Concepts of Health Promotion and Disease Prevention and how to use them in clinical practice. I shall do this by considering at some length the definitions of the basic terms in the field of health promotion/disease prevention.

A. DIFFERENT USES OF THE TERM

Health, as well as *disease*, *illness*, and *wellness* are terms we often use without considering their precise definitions. Over time many have been offered (Arnold and Breen, 1998; Downie, Tannahill, & Tannahill, 1996). It is easy to think of health simply as being the absence of disease, as well as to think of illness and disease as being interchangeable terms. In fact, health and disease are not simply opposites, and disease and illness do not mean the same thing (Downie, et al., 1996; Kass, 1981; Wolinsky, 1988).

Complicating matters further, in many of our uses of the word *health* we are not actually referring to any true aspect of health in virtually any sense of the term. For example, the word health is often used as an adjective when by no definition is health the focus of what is being described. Thus, what we often call "health statistics" are in fact disease statistics, and "health care," certainly in the Western approach, is in fact most often disease care. Jago (1975) listed 43 examples of such use, including the terms "health status," "health center," and "health worker." In practice, these most often mean, respectively, "sickness status," "disease treatment center," and "disease care worker."

B. THE GREEK VIEW

The consideration of just what health is has a long history and a wide geographic distribution. The ancient Greeks made a philosophic distinction between the concepts of health and disease. As the eminent medical historian Henry Sigerist (1941) said:

> The [Greek] physicians had an explanation for health. Health, they believed, was a condition of perfect equilibrium. When the forces or humors or whatever constituted the human body were perfectly balanced, man was healthy. Disturbed balance resulted in disease. This is still the best general explanation we have. (p. 57)

And it is the source of Concept VII, below.

What Dr. Sigerist described was not the position taken by all Greek physicians, however. It was the view of the followers of the Greek goddess of health, Hygeia, daughter of Apollo the supreme healer (Durant, 1939, pp. 342–348). The Greek physician Hippocrates, for whom the present professional oath that many medical school graduates take is named, focussed much of his own teaching on health promotion. For the individual, he addressed such elements as exercise, nutrition, and the active application of the "Greek mean," that is, moderation in all things, to achieve the desired balance in life. For the population as a whole, Hippocrates' teachings addressed public health measures to the extent they were understood at the time.

In contrast with the *hygienists*, followers of the Greek god of medicine, Asklepios (a son of Apollo) concentrated on disease and miracle cures. It is interesting to note that while both Hygeia and Asklepios were children of Apollo, it was the female who focussed on health while the male focussed on disease. Thinking of the principal philosophic base of male-dominated Western medicine as contrasted with that of female-dominated nursing, how marvelously modern that distinction is!

The Romans continued the Greek "Hygienic" approach to health, stressing its public health aspects especially. However, with the collapse of civilization that accompanied the gradual disintegration of the Roman Empire and the eventual rise of Christianity, in Europe the interest in disease almost entirely displaced any interest in the Greek idea of health. The concept of health, for example, as a state of optimal balance, would have little meaning either to the disease-wracked populace living in Europe from the Dark Ages through the Enlightenment, or to the practitioners of one kind or another who attempted to take care of them.

Magic and religious salvation, on the one hand, and on the other, miracle cures (and later) the early stages of scientifically based treatment of any departure from health after it became apparent, became the focus of what attention to health there was. As is well known, in contemporary Western medicine treating departures from health after they occur, the Asklepian (Aesculapian in Latin) approach, still receives most of the attention, in contrast with the Greco-Roman hygienic approach.

C. THE MODERN WESTERN APPROACH

In our own era, even after the vast development of science-based medicine, the idea of an approach to health based on curing, even of miracle cures (think of the term "medical miracle" often applied to the latest surgical or pharmaceutical intervention appearing on the scene) has persisted. It is still a seductive dream. Cures are sought that can compensate, not for unknown or misunderstood causes of illness, not just for causes of illness and injury beyond anyone's control, but also for well-known abuses of the body the individual and society have themselves perpetrated.

The desire of the developers of this group of cures is to be able to correct at a stroke, in full or in part, the effects of cigarette smoking, or eating an unhealthy diet, or working in an unhealthy work-place, or living in a highly stressful environment, over a period of years. This is the case even when prevention would be much more effective in promoting health than treatment would be, to say nothing of being much cheaper. For many Western health professionals it seems to be easier to care for disease than to promote good health. Moreover, for many, health promotion/disease prevention (HP/DP) lacks the drama associated with the high-technology crisis care so often observed in many of our hospitals (as well as on most of our medical drama TV shows).

Turning to contemporary definitions of health, despite the emphasis on curing characteristic of Western health care delivery systems, stepping across both geographic and historic boundaries, the World Health Organization (WHO) has adopted a definition of health that resonates much more with Hygeia than with Asklepios. For the WHO (1985) health is "a state of complete physical, mental, and social well-being, and not merely the absence of disease or infirmity" (p. 459).

This definition obviously reflects the Hygienic notion that health is a positive state. It is interesting to note how the WHO approach reflects the thinking of non-Western cultures.

D. SOME NON-WESTERN APPROACHES

Sidney Kark (1974), the South African/Israeli epidemiologist, quoted a Hindu physician thusly, "To the Hindu, health is harmony; [harmony is] being at peace with the Self, the community, God and the cosmos" (p. 11).

This idea comprehends both balance with the outside world and balance within the person, as necessary for the achievement and maintenance of health. The Taoist concept of health is much the same (Cohen, 1998). Kark, quoting Adair and Deuschle, also cited the Navajo concept of health. The similarities to the Eastern philosophies cited are striking:

[When there is] balance between the individual and his total physical and social environment, as well as . . . balance between the supernatural and man . . . good health is the result; and upset in this equilibrium causes disease. (p. 11)

How like those of the Greek followers of Hygeia these thoughts are (and again see Concept VII).

E. APPROACHING A COMPREHENSIVE DEFINITION

In general, modern Western definitions of health do not give balance pride of place, to say the least. For example, *The Random House Dictionary of the English Language, Second Edition, Unabridged* defines health in part by its supposed relationship to disease (Flexner, 1987). Health first is characterized as "the general condition of the body or mind with reference to soundness or vigor," but also as, "freedom from disease or ailment." Disease, too, *The Random House Dictionary* defines in part by citing the supposed opposite of health: "a disordered or incorrectly functioning organ, part, structure or system of the body. . . ."

The WHO definition (see above) has been criticized as being utopian (Dubos, 1971; Kass, 1981). A more functional definition is that proposed by Kass, namely, "the well-working of the organism as a whole" (p. 4). Other definitions of health, too, have stressed life functioning, for example seeing health as the "state of optimum capacity for effective performance of valued tasks" (Parsons, 1958, p. 168) or as "personal fitness for survival and self-renewal, creative social adjustment, and self-fulfillment" (Hoyman, 1967, p. 189).

The 1988 (international) *Consensus Statement on Exercise, Fitness, and Health* defined health as (Bouchard, Shepard, & Stephens):

. . . a human condition with physical, social, and psychological dimensions, each characterized on a continuum with positive and negative poles. Positive health is associated with a capacity to enjoy life and to withstand challenges; it is not merely the absence of disease. Negative health is associated with morbidity and, in the extreme, with premature mortality." (p. 84)

Included in a comprehensive definition of health promotion developed for the *American Journal of Health Promotion* (O'Donnell,

1989; for further discussion see chapter 3) is the following: "Optimal health is defined as a balance of physical, emotional, social, spiritual and intellectual health."

Taking into account all of these different approaches to a definition of health and many others not quoted here, a useful functional definition of health is perhaps this one:

> Health is a positive, balanced, state of being characterized by the best achievable physical, psychological, emotional, social, spiritual, and intellectual levels of functioning at a given time, the absence of disease or the optimal management of chronic disease, and the control of both internal and external risk factors* for both diseases and negative health conditions.

This is the definition comprehended by Concept I (*see* chapter 4). Common to virtually all of the definitions presented is that health is indeed a state of being, and a measurable one at that.

II. THE PURPOSE OF BEING HEALTHY

Regardless of the definition of health one might choose to use, what does health do for us? There are almost as many views on this question as there are definitions of health. For example, Herophilus, an ancient Greek physician who lived in Alexandria, Egypt, said:

> When health is absent, wisdom cannot reveal itself, art cannot become manifest, strength cannot fight, wealth becomes useless, and intelligence cannot be applied. (Sigerist, 1941, p. 57)

In 1787, Thomas Jefferson, who addressed so many subjects with so much wisdom, wrote:

> Without health there is no happiness. And attention to health, then, should take the place of every other object. The time necessary to secure this by active exercises should be devoted to it in preference to every other pursuit. I know the difficulty with which

---

* A risk factor is some environmental element, personal habit, or condition of living that increases the likelihood of developing a particular disease or negative health condition at some time in the future.

a strenuous man tears himself from his studies at any given moment of the day; but his happiness, and that of his family depend on it. The most uninformed mind, with a healthy body, is happier than the wisest valetudinarian [person in poor health]. (Foley, 1967, p. 402)

The late, great "running doctor" George Sheehan (1989), put it in a slightly simpler way, "Health makes for the happy pursuit of happiness and gives us a longer time to do it" (p. 24).

As Breslow (1996) said, "[E]xpanding people's capacity to extend enjoyable life . . . constitutes health."

III. DEFINITIONS OF DISEASE AND ILLNESS

While they are not the opposites of health, disease and illness are certainly in the same ballpark with it. A classic medical dictionary, *Blakiston's* (1956), took a precise, functional approach to defining disease:

a failure of the adaptive mechanisms of an organism to counter-act adequately the stimuli and stresses to which it is subject, result-ing in a disturbance in function or structure of any part, organ, or system of the body.

Like *Blakiston's*, the *Random House Unabridged Dictionary* (Flexner, 1987) is precise:

a disordered or incorrectly functioning organ, part, structure, or system of the body resulting from the effect of genetic or devel-opmental errors, infection, poisons, nutritional deficiency or imbal-ance, toxicity, or unfavorable environmental factors. . .

Whatever its definition, however, disease is a biomedical concept. Disease is something that a health care worker finds. Illness, on the other hand, is a state of being; it is something the ill person feels (Downie, et al., 1996, pp. 10–12). As Eric Cassell (1976) once said:

. . . let us use the word "illness" to stand for what the patient feels when he goes to the doctor and "disease" for what he has on the

way home from the doctor's office. Disease, then, is something
an organ has; illness is something a man has. (p. 48)

Illness thus has social and psychological as well as biomedical
components. One can have a disease without feeling ill, as in asymp-
tomatic cancer; and one can surely feel ill without being diseased.

IV. SOME SOCIAL FACTORS IN HEALTH AND ILLNESS

Illness can be seen both as a biologic phenomenon and as a social
role (sometimes called the "sick role") that carries with it certain
rights and obligations (Brown, 1989, pp. 142–145). Further, some illnesses are at least in part self-induced. However, even when a person *seems* to have brought an illness on oneself—as in a personal
injury resulting from carelessness or lung cancer caused by cigarette smoking—we now know that rarely are they solely responsible for their condition (Breslow, 1996).

For example, the seriousness of a personal injury arising from a
given automobile collision, even when one is driving drunk, is often
influenced by external factors, such as, the presence or absence of
airbags in the automobile. Whether or not to smoke cigarettes is an
individual decision. But in the overwhelming majority of cases that
decision is made during the preteen or teen-age years, when a person is most susceptible to both tobacco company advertising and
the relatively infinite availability of cigarette supply at relatively
low prices. Nicotine in cigarettes is a highly addictive drug. Then
once hooked, smokers are subject to the continuous manipulation
of nicotine levels in cigarettes by the tobacco companies (*Tobacco on
Trial*).

Thus going beyond the individual to society as a whole, it is by
now clear that social factors have a very significant impact on disease and health (Brown, 1989). Although much remains to be
learned, the science of social epidemiology (Wolinsky, 1988) has elu
cidated the relationship between states of health and illness and
many social/societal characteristics.

These include nationality, social class, race, employment status,
occupation, behavior patterns, societal promotion of illness (by, for
example, the tobacco companies), societal promotion of prevention

(by, for example, governmental requirements for safe automobile design), and geography. It is the strategies of social ecology that attempt to influence this concatenation of health influences at the societal level in a positive direction (Breslow, 1996).

V. DEFINITIONS AND DESCRIPTIONS OF WELLNESS

Halbert Dunn, a retired Public Health Service physician, developed the concept of what he called "high-level wellness." For the individual he defined it as (Dunn, 1961/1977):

> an integrated method of functioning which is oriented toward maximizing the potential of which the individual is capable. It requires that the individual maintain a continuum of balance and purposeful direction within the environment where he is functioning. (p. 4)

This approach emphasizes the incorporation of good health habits into one's everyday life (Gorin & Arnold, 1998; Jonas & Konner, 1997; Kassberg & Jonas, 1999). We shall in this book use Dr. Dunn's definition of "high-level wellness" as our primary one for "wellness," unmodified. At the same time, it is useful to consider several other related definitions and descriptions of the meaning of the term that have been put forward.

For example, Dunn himself elaborated on his concept, stating that "wellness is a direction in progress toward an ever-higher potential of functioning" (p. 6). One of the principal proponents of the concept of wellness during the last quarter of the twentieth century has been Dr. Don Ardell. He has offered a variety of (closely related) definitions of wellness.

For example, in 1984 he said that wellness is

> [A] conscious and deliberate approach to an advanced state of physical and psychological/spiritual health. This is a dynamic or ever-changing, fluctuating state of being. (Ardell, 1984, p. 5)

Ardell (1986) further defined the concept as:

> giving care to the physical self, using the mind constructively, channeling stress energies positively, expressing emotions effec-

tively, becoming creatively involved with others, and staying in touch with the environment.

He also said that:

In pursuing wellness . . . your mind, body, and spirit are integrated and inseparable . . . the total *you* must be involved, including your self-concept, your work, your primary and other relationships, your environment, and so forth. (1986, p. 55; quotation slightly reordered)

Ten years later he said:

Wellness is essentially a lifestyle that encompasses a set of principles, such as the belief in the values of making thoughtful, disciplined choices with respect to such issues as exercise and nutrition. It entails skills, such as a capacity for managing stress and functioning with a commitment to embracing personal as well as social responsibility. And, not last and surely not least, wellness can and must lead to a lifelong quest for insights and understanding, satisfaction, and excitement for the greatest quest of all, namely, making wise decisions about life's Meaning and Purposes.

In summary, wellness offers those who seek to create their own form of a good life (rather than passively hoping it will happen) a broad set of guides for high levels of being. It is a concept for improving the chances for realizing and enjoying exceptional health. It promotes your chances for a satisfying and fulfilling life perceived as meaningful and filled with worthy purposes. (1996, pp. 69–70)

Continuing to explore the concept, from the level of nuance to the level of grand design, in 1998 Ardell further defined wellness as follows:

Wellness . . . is devoted to the promotion of a strategy or philosophy that will help you achieve an optimal level of physical and psychological well-being AND enjoy a wonderfully successful and satisfying life of consequence. (1998b)

Recently, Ardell has also placed wellness into the broad political context, relating it to the basic precepts of the Declaration of Independence and the Constitution of the United States including the Bill of Rights (Ardell, 1998a, c).

In 1999, he continued in this vein. In the 53rd edition of the *Ardell Wellness Report* (1999), he answered his own rhetorical question, "What is Wellness?" by saying, in part:

> Wellness is about perspective, about balance and about the big picture. It is a lifestyle and a personalized approach to living your life in such a way that you enjoy maximum freedom, including freedom FROM illness/disability and premature death to the extent possible, and freedom TO experience life, liberty and the pursuit of happiness. It is a declaration of independence for becoming the best kind of person that your potentials, circumstances and fate will allow." (p. 1)

Putting these thoughts together, we can see that wellness is a life-long *process* of striving towards a *state* of health. (Recall that the idea that "health" is a state of being—and one that is measurable—appears in virtually all of the definitions offered in the first section of this chapter.) Encompassing all the elements of living, for the well person the process ends only with death or an unmodifiable prelude to it: The terminal condition. Wellness is thus a journey that has many intermediate milestones but no final endpoints.

Central to the concept of wellness is recognizing that what constitutes a "personal state of well-being" for any individual can vary over time. In most of us, it does indeed vary over time. As Ardell (1986) succinctly put it, "Don't Sacrifice, Deny Yourself, or give Up Destructive Life Habits—Until You're Ready to Do So" (p. 52)

Finally on the concept of wellness, there is the question: are prevention, health, and wellness in different arenas, concerned with vastly different aspects of living? In describing his newsletter, *The Ardell Wellness Report*, Ardell (1999) does see a contradiction between traditional disease prevention/health promotion on the one hand and wellness on the other:

> This is a wellness newsletter—REAL wellness, not that sissy stuff you find in medical[ly] oriented[,] prevention[-] dominated[,] health education stuff. [This] is wellness beyond just health.

But if health is a state of being and wellness a process of being—recall that Dunn described the latter as "a direction in progress toward an ever-higher potential of functioning," and note that Ardell's own definitions reflect the same understanding—then prevention, health, and wellness are not mutually exclusive. Rather, they are all part of that complex, dynamic, three-dimensional feedback loop referred to in chapter 1.

In each of us, disease prevention, health promotion, and wellness, if undertaken positively in a balanced manner, are continually serving to enhance both our health (status) and our wellness (process). For the healthier one is, the more capable one is of being well, and the more well one is, the better is one equipped to be and stay healthy.

If wellness is The Way, then even "medically oriented, prevention-dominated, health education stuff"—promoting health by, say risk-factor reduction and early disease-detection—can be seen as two of the (although certainly not the only) engines, and powerful engines at that, that we can use to motor on it.

VI. GETTING ON THE WELLNESS ROAD

How then do we get on the wellness road and stay there? Dr. William Hettler of the National Wellness Institute and the University of Wisconsin at Stevens Point, one of the early developers of campus wellness programs, modifying early work of Ardell (1986) that proposed a list of "dimensions," or one might say "realms," of wellness came up with six groups of components: "Occupational, Vocational; Physical Fitness, Nutrition; Emotional; Social, Family, Community, Environmental; Intellectual; Spiritual, Values, Ethics" (pp. 324–326).

Note that in this list are several elements not usually associated with health, but often associated with wellness: the intellectual, the cultural, and the spiritual dimensions or realms of life.

At the State University of New York at Stony Brook, Marcia Wiener, Peter Mastroianni, and their colleagues at The Eugene Weidman Wellness Center and on the Campus-Wide Wellness Program Planning Committee have developed their own adaptation of the work of Hettler and the National Wellness Institute on the dimensions of wellness (Weidman Wellness Center). They call their approach "Centering." This is another term for "Achieving Balance," the "Dynamic Goal" of Concept VII (see chapter 3). The approach is visually represented as the Center's "Wellness Wheel," having eight components (Weidman Wellness Center): "Get Centered! Physically, emotionally, intellectually, environmentally, culturally, occupationally, spiritually, and socially."

Recently a ninth component, creativity, has been added. The definitions for the nine components follow.

Physical. The physical dimension encourages physical activity that promotes cardiovascular fitness, flexibility, and strength. Physical development encourages fitness and a healthy eating pattern based on food and nutrition knowledge, includes medical self-care and appropriate use of the medical and holistic health systems. The use of tobacco and other drugs is inconsistent with a wellness lifestyle. Alcohol in particular, should be avoided or used in moderation and greater understanding and care taken when using prescription medications, homeopathic remedies, herbs, or dietary supplements.

Emotional. The emotional dimension emphasizes an awareness and acceptance of one's feelings. Emotional wellness includes the degree to which one feels positive and enthusiastic about oneself and life. It includes the capacity to manage one's feelings and related behaviors including the realistic assessment of one's limitations, development of autonomy, and ability to cope effectively with stress. The emotionally well person maintains satisfying relationships with others.

Intellectual. The intellectual dimension encourages creative, stimulating mental activities. An intellectually well person uses the resources available to expand one's knowledge and improve skills, along with expanding potential for sharing with others. An intellectually well person uses the intellectual and cultural activities both in the classroom and beyond the classroom, combined with the human resources and learning resources available both within the university community and the larger community.

Environmental. The environmental dimension explores the world we live in seeking harmony with our surroundings. An environmentally well person aims toward a balance between human needs and environmental needs and takes action to protect and preserve the natural world. Finding time on a regular basis to enjoy contact with nature is also an important component of a wellness lifestyle.

Cultural. The cultural dimension emphasizes an awareness, acceptance, and appreciation for diverse cultures and backgrounds as well as understanding and valuing one's own culture. A culturally well person understands that through interaction with other groups, knowledge will be achieved and respect developed.

Occupational. The occupational dimension is involved in preparing and utilizing one's gifts, skills, and talents in order to gain personal purpose, satisfaction, and enrichment in one's life. This allows one to maintain a positive attitude and experience satisfaction and pleasure in one's work.

Spiritual. The spiritual dimension involves seeking meaning and purpose in one's life. It includes the development of a deep appreciation for human experience and diversity of spiritual expression. Spiritual growth includes a strengthening of our connection with others and increased recognition of, and appreciation for, our own ability to affect the world in a positive way.

Social. The social dimension encourages contributing to one's human and physical environment to the common welfare of one's community. It emphasizes the interdependence with others. It includes the pursuit of harmony in one's family and all communities in which one interacts. It also entails protecting oneself from unhealthy relationships, and learning to build healthy ones based on trust, respect, and open communication. Healthy relationships help a person feel good about themselves while unhealthy ones have the opposite effect.

Creative. The creative dimension is best illustrated by a child's wonderment of their world, the human need to explore and the desire to seek proficiency in adapting to that world. One is developing within this dimension whenever they are engaged in the processes of building, creating, improving, discovering, solving, planning, dancing, drawing, painting sculpting, acting. The common process in all of these is drawing from within, using your feelings and intelligence in the process.

Finally, it must be noted that as we get on the wellness road or pathway or journey we must recall that it is a journey without end. Wellness, we must repeat, is a process of being, not a state of being. Furthermore, wellness and the striving for it must be seen as facilitating a better life, not as creating for us a series of hurdles that must be overcome. Above all, on the wellness road one must not be caught up in perfectionism. For humans, perfection is impossible to achieve. Perfection*ism* is therefore a destructive process. Another way of putting it is to say: "We can never be perfect; we can always get better."

REFERENCES

Ardell, D. B. (1984). *The history and future of wellness.* Pleasant Hill, CA: Diablo Press.

Ardell, D. B. (1986). *High level wellness: An alternative to doctors, drugs, and disease.* Berkeley, CA: Ten Speed Press.

Ardell, D. B. (1996). *The book of wellness: A secular approach to spirit, meaning & purpose.* Amherst, NY: Prometheus Books.

Ardell, D. B. (1998a, Summer). The History of Wellness. *Ardell Wellness Report, 50,* 3.

Ardell, D. B. (1998b, September 16). Ask the Wellness Expert from the show "Ask the Wellness Expert," *www.yourhealth.com*

Ardell, D. B. (1998c, October 6). Declaration of Independence and Wellness, from the show "Ask the Wellness Expert," *www. yourhealth.com*

Ardell, D. B. (1999, Summer). "What is Wellness" *Ardell Wellness Report, 53,* 1.

Arnold, J., & Breen, L. J. (1998). Images of Health. In S. S. Gorin, & J. Arnold. *Health promotion handbook.* St. Louis, MO: Mosby.

Blakiston's new gould medical dictionary (2nd ed) (1956). New York: Blakiston Division, McGraw-Hill.

Bouchard, C., Shepard, R. J., & Stephens, T. (Eds.). (1988). *Physical activity, fitness, and health: International proceedings and consensus statement.* Champaign, IL: Human Kinetics Publishers.

Breslow, L. (1996). Social Ecological Strategies for Promoting Healthy Lifestyles. *American Journal of Health Promotion, 10,* 253.

Brown, P. (Ed.). (1989). *Perspectives in medical sociology,* Blooming, CA: Wadsworth.

Cassell, E. (1976). *The healer's art.* Philadelphia: Lippincott.

Cohen, K. (1998). *Taoism: Study guide.* Boulder, CO: Sounds True.

Downie, R.S., Tannahill, C., & Tannahill, A. (1996). *Health promotion: Models and values.* Oxford, England: Oxford University Press.

Dubos, R. (1971). *Mirage of health.* New York: Harper & Row.

Dunn, H. L., *High-level wellness.* (1961/1977). Thorofare, NJ: Charles B. Slack.

Durant, W. (1939). *The life of Greece.* New York: Simon and Schuster.

Flexner, S. B. (Ed.). (1987). *The Random House dictionary of the English language, 2nd edition unabridged,* New York: Random House.

Foley, J. P. (Ed.). (1967). *Jeffersonian cyclopedia: A comprehensive collection of the views of Thomas Jefferson* (Vol. I). New York: Russell and Russell.

Gorin, S. S., & Arnold, J. (1998). *Health promotion handbook.* St. Louis, MO: Mosby.

Hoyman, H. (1967). The Spiritual Dimensions of Man's Health in Today's World. In D. Belgum (Ed.), *Religion and medicine.* Ames, IA: Iowa State University Press.

Jago, J. (1975). "Health"—Old word, new task: Refections on the words "Health" and "Medical". *Social Science and Medicine, 9,* 1.

Jonas, S., & Konner, L. (1997). *Just the weigh you are: How to be fit and healthy, whatever your size.* Boston, MA: Chapters Publishing/ Houghton/Mifflin.

Kark, S. (1974). *Epidemiology and community medicine.* New York: Appleton-Century-Crofts.

Kass, L. (1981). Regarding the end of medicine and the pursuit of health. In A. Caplan, H. T. Engelhardt, & J. McCartney (Eds.), *Concepts of health and disease, interdisciplinary perspectives,* (pp. 3–30). Reading, MA: Addison-Wesley.

Kassberg, M., & Jonas, S. (1999). *Help your man get healthy: An essentiul guide for every caring woman.* New York: Whole Care/Avon Books.

O'Donnell, M. P. (1989). Definition of Health Promotion: Part III: Expanding the Definition. *American Journal of Health Promotion, 3,* 5.

Parsons, T. (1958). Definitions of Health and Illness in the Light of American Values and Social Structure. In E. Jaco (Ed.), *Patients, physicians, and illness.* Glencoe, IL: The Free Press.

Sigerist, H. (1941). *Medicine and human welfare.* New Haven, CT: Yale University Press.

Tobacco on Trial, "A Drug is a Drug," October, 1995, p. 1.

Weidman Wellness Center, (1998). [Brochure] Stony Brook, NY: State University of New York at Stony Brook.

Wolinsky, F. D. (1988). *The sociology of health*. Belmont, CA: Wadsworth
    Publishing Co.
World Health Organization. (1958). *The World Health Organization: A
    report on the first ten years*. Geneva, Switzerland: Author.

Chapter 3

WHY HEALTH PROMOTION/ DISEASE PREVENTION?

I. WHAT ARE HEALTH PROMOTION AND DISEASE PREVENTION?

A. HEALTH PROMOTION

An important program element in helping people get on the well-ness pathway is that set of activities known as "Health Promotion." Downie, Tannahill, and Tannahill (1996) have considered the term and what it means at some length. First, they offer the following warning to those exploring its meaning:

> [I]t is most unfortunate that [the term] "health promotion" is used in a number of different ways, even by the same people. . . . In effect, health promotion has become a dazzling band-wagon, gain-ing momentum, and with all and sundry clamouring to climb aboard, without giving sufficient thought to where it is going. (pp. 56–61)

However, using a model developed by one of them (Tannahill, 1985), they go on to offer the following comprehensive definition:

[H]ealth promotion comprises three overlapping spheres of activity: *health education** (or, more precisely, that part which contributes to the overall goal of health promotion), *prevention*, and *health protection*. (1996, p. 58)

They identify the following domains of health promotion:

- Preventive measures such as immunization and cervical screening.
- Educational efforts to influence lifestyle in the interests of preventing ill-health, as well as efforts to encourage the uptake of preventive services.
- Preventive health protection" (such as the fluoridation of water, communicable disease control, and occupational health and safety).
- Education of policy-makers.
- Health education aimed at influencing behaviour on positive health grounds . . . and that which seeks to help individuals, groups, or whole communities to develop positive health attributes.
- Raising awareness of, and securing support for, positive health protection measures, among the public and policy-makers. (pp. 59–60)

They then arrive at a brief but comprehensive definition of health promotion:

Health promotion comprises efforts to enhance positive health and reduce the risk of ill-health, through the overlapping spheres of health education, prevention, and health protection. (p. 60)

The American authority on health, Lester Breslow (1996), cites the brief definition developed by the First International Conference on Health Promotion, found in the "Ottawa Charter for Health

---

* In turn, Downie, Tannahill, and Tannahill (1996) define health education as a system that "seeks to enhance positive health and to prevent or diminish ill-health, through influencing beliefs, attitudes, and behaviour. The stimulation of a healthful environment—social and political as well as physical—is an important objective" (p. 48).

Promotion": "[Health promotion is] the process of enabling people to increase control over, and to improve, their own health" (p. 253).

Dr. Michael O'Donnell and colleagues developed a very useful definition of health promotion for the *American Journal of Health Promotion* (O'Donnell, 1989; the sentence defining "health" is referred to in chapter 1):

> Health promotion is the science and art of helping people change their lifestyle to move toward a state of optimal health. Optimal health is defined as a balance of physical, emotional, social, spiritual and intellectual health. Lifestyle change can be facilitated through a combination of efforts to enhance awareness, change behavior and create environments that support good health practices. Of the three, supportive environments will probably have the greatest impact in producing lasting change.

This is the working definition used for this book. (It is interesting to note the emphasis given to the importance of environmental factors by both O'Donnell and colleagues and, in their definition of health education [see footnote], Downie and colleagues. See also, Breslow, in chapter 5.)

B. DISEASE PREVENTION

Downie and colleagues (1996) have also considered the definition of prevention. They note that:

> Central to prevention is the notion of reducing the risk of occurrence of a disease process, illness, injury, disability, handicap, or some other unwanted phenomenon or state. (pp. 50–52)

Three levels of prevention can be identified: primary, secondary, and tertiary. Primary prevention is stopping disease before it starts, as in immunization against an infectious disease, preventing a child from commencing to smoke cigarettes, or helping an adult to stop smoking cigarettes before the onset of any of the myriad diseases and negative health conditions associated with that addiction that is so heavily promoted by its purveyors in the tobacco industry.

Secondary prevention is the early detection of existing disease before it becomes clinically apparent, as in screening for hypertension or various forms of cancer. Tertiary prevention is the optimum management of clinically apparent disease so as to prevent or at least minimize the development of future complications, as in the control of blood sugar level in diabetes mellitus.

Each of these levels of prevention can appear in each of the classes of health service: the "personal," the "community," and the "combined" (for the definitions of these terms see below under the section on the role of the health care delivery system, pp. 35ff).

II. THE POWER OF HEALTH PROMOTION AND DISEASE PREVENTION

One way to gain an appreciation for the power of health promotion and disease prevention to improve the health of both individuals and populations in the United States is to examine the leading causes of death for their relative preventability. The customary way to do this has been to use for the rankings the disease-specific causes of death found on death certificates, such as heart disease, cancer, and stroke.

There is a newer approach to the subject, much more useful than the traditional one when planning approaches to health promotion and disease prevention programs for both individuals and populations. It is to rank the numbers of deaths as they are associated with the major environmental/behavioral risk factors linked to (premature) death, for example, cigarette smoking, unhealthy eating patterns, and sedentary lifestyle. Most of the listed risk factors are associated with a number of different major killer diseases.

This risk-factor approach is much more patient/client-centered than the traditional disease-oriented one. For patients and clients come to health care providers for the most part not with, for example, a "prevent a heart attack" need but rather with a "help me to stop smoking" need. Understanding the difference between medically defined causes of death and real-time factors that increase the risk of premature, painful, debilitating, slow, death is very important for effective health promotion/disease prevention (HP/DP) intervention.

As of 1997, the top 10 causes of death by medical diagnosis in the United States were: heart disease, cancer, stroke, chronic obstructive pulmonary disease, personal injury, pneumonia and influenza, diabetes mellitus, suicide, kidney disease, chronic liver disease and cirrhosis (Hoyert, Kochanek, & Murphy, 1999). This way of categorizing causes of death originated hundreds of years ago. With the possible exception of kidney disease, the risk of occurrence at any given time of all of these diseases can be reduced, to a greater or lesser extent, by the use of appropriate HP/DP interventions.

When risk factors rather than medically defined diseases are used to quantify causes of death, the case for the power of HP/DP becomes even more impressive than it is just intuitively (as in "an ounce of prevention is worth a pound of cure"). In 1993, Drs. Michael McGinniss and William Foege for the first time in this country took the "other cut" on causes of death (McGinniss & Foege). They went beyond the classic lists of disease-specific numbers of death to the identification of the major external (that is, nongenetic) factors known to be causally associated with death. After an exhaustive review of the literature covering the period 1977–1993, they found that for 1991 approximately one half of all deaths could be attributed to the following *risk factors*:

- Tobacco use: 400,000 deaths
- Diet and activity patterns: 300,000 deaths
- Alcohol use: 100,000 deaths
- Microbial agents: 90,000 deaths
- Toxic agents: 60,000 deaths
- Firearms: 35,000 deaths
- Sexual behaviors: 30,000 deaths
- Motor vehicle use: 25,000 deaths
- Use of heroin, cocaine, and other "illicit" drugs: 20,000 deaths

As ballpark figures at least, it is likely that these numbers will continue to be obtained into the early twenty first century, at least.

The picture arising from the McGinniss and Foege analysis is particularly helpful in planning clinical HP/DP programs to prolong healthy life. These risk factors are all modifiable using known HP/DP interventions. In clinical practice, because, as mentioned, otherwise healthy patients/clients present primarily with risk factors, focussing on the related modifiable behaviors has much more relevance to them than does focussing on disease-defined proximate causes of death.

However, either way of organizing and listing the major causes of death shows that HP/DP have an enormous potential for improving the health of the American people. HP/DP program implementation can do this by both postponing death and increasing the number of years of life lived healthily before death inevitably occurs. As Wynder and Kristein said some time ago, in brief the primary goal of health promotion/disease prevention is to "help people die young—late in life" (1977).

The risk-factor modification approach is at the heart of the *"Healthy People"* program of the US Department of Health and Human Services (United States Department of Health and Human Services, 1991, 1995, 1998b, 1999) (see below, pp. 38ff). It is also at the center of the Behavioral Risk Factor Surveillance System of the Centers for Disease Control (*Morbidity and Mortality Weekly Report*, 1997).

III. THE ROLE OF MEDICINE IN IMPROVING HEALTH LEVELS OVER TIME

Despite the evidence on both the potential and actual power of prevention, many providers in our health care delivery system maintain the view that it is clinical medicine that is primarily responsible for the observed improvements in population health levels that have taken place over time.

It is certainly true that in our own era of science-based medicine on the clinical side very significant technological advances have been made in the measurement and visualization of internal body functioning, anesthesia, surgery, and pharmaceutical therapeutics. Thus, many people have the natural tendency to think that our collection of "modern medical miracles" has had a major positive impact on the population's health and its measures. However, while modern medicine has had a positive impact on many individual lives, interestingly enough it has had little impact on health as it is measured in populations. Consider the following evidence.

In 1857 the tuberculosis death rate in Massachusetts was 450 per 100,000; by 1890, the rate had fallen to 250; by 1920, to 114; and by 1938, to 35.6 (Sigerist, 1941, p. 46). Yet the first effective therapy for tuberculosis, the antibiotic streptomycin (succeeded quickly by other drugs when its tendency to produce deafness in longer-term users was noted) was not available for general use until 1948. Why the dramatic decline in the tuberculosis death rate before that date, without the direct intervention of effective medical care? The strong likelihood is that it was almost entirely related to environmental factors.

In the 1970s, Prof. Thomas McKeown of the University of Birmingham (England) examined this observed phenomenon in great detail (1976; 1997). His analysis of falling overall death rates and increasing population size from 1841 in England and Wales showed that these changes preceded the introduction of any effective direct medical intervention by a considerable period of time. The overall death rate in England and Wales fell from about 22 per 1000 in 1841 to around 6 per 1000 in 1971. In his seminal study, Prof. McKeown was able to show that 92% of the death rate decline between 1848 and 1901 and 73% of that between 1901 and 1971 resulted from a reduction in the number of deaths from infectious diseases (1976, pp. 93–94).

He began his analysis by taking a close look at death rates for England and Wales over time. He found that most of the overall death rate reduction was due to a drop in the tuberculosis death rate that paralleled the one that occurred in Massachusetts during the same period. As was the case in Massachusetts, in England and Wales death rates from respiratory tuberculosis fell steadily from 1838, although, as noted above, effective chemotherapy for the disease was not available until 1948.

This is not to say that chemotherapy, for tuberculosis and many other illnesses, has not saved many lives and made countless others more comfortable, as likewise have many other modern medical advances. Nor is it to say that effective treatments should not be sought. After 1948, the decline in the tuberculosis death rate did accelerate further from the relatively low point it had already reached, indicating a positive effect of chemotherapy.

Nor is it to say that all these discoveries and interventions should not have been made because their results have little impact on population health data. It is to say precisely that the fact that the many "medical miracles" don't show up as having much impact on population health data, while various health promotive/disease preventive measures do, informs the focus of this book on personal HP/DP.

To further strengthen his case, McKeown also examined the historic changes in the death rates for bronchitis, pneumonia, and influenza. After tuberculosis, they were the major causes of mortality during the infectious disease era. It turned out that the death rates for these conditions were also little affected by the introduction of antibiotics. As was the case with tuberculosis, they had dropped significantly before the advent of the antibiotic era.

McKeown then examined the factors that could possibly have accounted for the observed changes. He concluded that the most important influence on the rising population health levels that occurred during that time was the large improvement in human nutrition that took place during the period 1750 to 1950. He concluded further that the first element in that improvement was simply a very significant increase in food supply. It resulted from several important technologic and ecologic changes: a major improvement in farming techniques, the development of the first bulk transportation system, the canals, and possibly the climatic warming trend that occurred just before the onset of the large increase in food production.

McKeown (1976) estimated that hygienic measures, such as the advent of clean water supply and sanitary sewage disposal, were responsible for about one fifth of the reduction in death rates. Moreover, he stated:

> With the exception of vaccination against smallpox, whose contribution was small, the influence of [primarily anti-viral] immunization and [anti-bacterial] therapy on the death rate was delayed until the 20th century, and had little effect on national mortality trends before the introduction of sulphonamides in 1935. Since that time it has not been the only, or [even] the most important influence. (p. 94)

Even in our own era, public health and preventive medicine measures continue to be primarily responsible for the observed reductions in mortality rates. For example, since the mid-1970s in the United States there have been significant declines in the heart disease, stroke, personal injury, and non-tobacco-related cancer death rates (McGinnis, 1990; MMWR, 1999b; USDHHS, 1998a).

It appears that these declines are again primarily the result of preventive measures such as improved early detection and treatment of hypertension, public health and law enforcement programs leading to the reduction in driving while intoxicated-related trauma and the increased use of automobile seat belts, and educational programs leading to the lowering of dietary fat intake and the decline in cigarette smoking among adults. The evidence supports the view that treatment, except as a concomitant of an intervention that is in the first instance preventive, such as screening, has had little impact on death rates.

IV. THE ROLE OF THE HEALTH CARE DELIVERY SYSTEM IN MODERN HEALTH PROMOTION/DISEASE PREVENTION

A. DEFINITIONS

The health care delivery system has been defined in terms of its components (Jonas, 1998):

> the health care institutions, the personnel who work in them, the firms producing "health commodities" such as pharmaceutical drugs and hospital equipment, the research and educational institutions that produce biomedical knowledge and health care personnel, and the financing mechanism. (p. 6)

Taking a less functional, more outcome-oriented viewpoint than any of the above, Weinerman (1971) defined the health care services system as:

> All of the activities of a society which are designed to protect or restore health, whether directed to the individual, the community, or the environment. (p. 273)

B. The Categories of Health Services

However they are defined, whatever emphasis may be given to one group or another, health services are conventionally divided into two broad categories: personal and community. Personal health services are those provided directly to individuals, for the maintenance of health and the control or cure of illness. Community health services are those provided to population groups. In many of the latter cases, members of the target population are unaware that the service is being provided unless there is some breakdown in it. Examples of community health services are the provision of pure water supply; sanitary sewage and solid waste disposal; toxic waste control; food, milk, and drug inspection and control; fluoridation of water; workplace health and safety measures; and control of air and noise pollution.

There is a third group of health services that can be identified: those that have aspects of both the community and personal health groups. They can be called "combined" services. For example, certain mass immunization programs protect both each immunized individual and the community as a whole through a phenomenon known as "herd immunity." This is especially the case for diseases caused by obligatory human parasites like the now-eradicated smallpox virus.* Other such combined community and individual services include tuberculosis and venereal disease case-finding and treatment programs, which while helping infected individuals also gradually reduce the total number of sources of infection for healthy persons, again producing herd immunity.

The importance of HP/DP for personal as well as community health in the twentieth century is reflected in the list of the "Ten Greatest Public Health Achievements—United States, 1900–1999" as determined by the *Morbidity and Mortality Weekly Report* published by the U.S. Centers for Disease Control and Prevention (April 2, 1999). They are:

---

* An obligatory human parasite is a microbe, like the smallpox virus, that, unlike the tetanus bacillus for example, cannot and does not survive outside of human beings. "Herd immunity" to infection develops when so few members of a given population are or can be infected with a given microbe that there is no longer a viable source of infection for that population as a whole.

- Vaccination
- Motor-vehicle safety
- Safer workplaces
- Control of infectious diseases
- Decline in deaths from coronary heart disease and stroke
- Safer and healthier foods
- Healthier mothers and babies
- Family planning
- Fluoridation of drinking water
- Recognition of tobacco use as a health hazard

There is, from one perspective, an even broader category of health service than community. If health care is in part aimed at improving or assisting social functioning, it must grapple with societal as well as individual or community-wide health problems. Perhaps overstating the case somewhat, Rudolph Virchow, the great German pathologist who as a youth in 1848 fought on the barricades against Bismarck's authoritarian Prussian government, described his profession in these words: "Medicine is a social science and politics is nothing else but medicine on a large scale" (Sigerist, 1941, p. 93)

V. HEALTH PROMOTION/DISEASE PREVENTION: THE BROADER CONTEXT

In 1979, the United States Public Health Service published *Healthy People: The Surgeon General's Report on Health Promotion and Disease Prevention* (United States Department of Health, Education, and Welfare, 1979). As the then Secretary of Department of Health, Education, and Welfare, Joseph Califano, said:

> . . . the purpose of this Report is to encourage a second public health revolution in the United States. . . . This document is properly optimistic about our growing scientific knowledge and about the possibility of setting clear measurable goals for public health action. (p. vii)

The *Report's* opening chapter states:

> It is the thesis of this report that further improvements in the health of the American people can and will be achieved—not through increased medical care and greater health expenditures—

but through a renewed national commitment to efforts designed
to prevent disease and to promote health. (p. 3)

The *Report* then set specific health objectives in 15 "priority areas"
for intervention, ranging from family planning and toxic agent control to smoking cessation. They were arranged in three categories:
Health Promotion, Health Protection, and Preventive Services.

In 1990, the Department of Health and Human Services published
the second iteration of this work, *Healthy People 2000: National Health
Promotion and Disease Prevention Objectives* (United States Department
of Health and Human Services, 1991). In his foreword to *Healthy
People 2000*, Dr. Louis Sullivan, then Secretary of Health and Human
Services, said:

. . . health promotion and disease prevention comprise perhaps
our best opportunity to reduce the ever-increasing portion of our
resources that we spend to treat preventable illness and functional
impairment. . . . We would be terribly remiss if we did not seize
the opportunity presented by health promotion and disease prevention to dramatically cut health care costs, to prevent the premature onset of disease and disability, and to help all Americans
achieve healthier, more productive lives.

Dr. Sullivan pointed out that illnesses related to cigarette smoking—a both preventable and treatable drug addiction—"cost our
health care system more than $65 billion annually [as of 1989]," that
AIDS, which in 10 years came from nowhere to be in the top 10
killers nationally, "is an almost entirely preventable disease," and
that alcoholism and drug abuse (other than cigarette smoking), both
significantly preventable, as of 1989 together cost the society over
$100 billion annually in treatment costs, premature death, personal
injury, crime, and lost productivity.

Continuing the emphasis of the original report, *Healthy People
2000* set three "overarching goals" (p. 43): increase the span of
healthy life for Americans, reduce health disparities among
Americans, achieve access to preventive services for all Americans.
To reach these goals, the number of "priority areas" for intervention was expanded to 22, grouped in the same intervention categories as presented in the 1979 *Report*, plus a new one for data
collection (Table 3.1).

Examples of objectives for the year 2000 included (pp. 91–125): Reduce coronary heart disease deaths to no more than 100 per 100,000 people; reduce deaths caused by unintentional injuries to no more than 29.3 per 100,000 people; increase years of healthy life

Table 3.1 National Health Promotion and Disease Prevention Objectives Priority Areas [for the Year 2000], Grouped by Category

Health Promotion
1. Physical activity and fitness
2. Nutrition
3. Tobacco
4. Substance abuse: alcohol and other drugs
5. Family Planning
6. Mental Health and Mental Disorders
7. Violent and Abusive Behavior
8. Educational and Community-Based Programs

Health Protection
9. Unintentional injuries
10. Occupational safety and health
11. Environmental health
12. Food and drug safety
13. Oral health

Preventive services
14. Maternal and infant health
15. Heart disease and stroke
16. Cancer
17. Diabetes and chronic disabling conditions
18. HIV infection
19. Sexually transmitted diseases
20. Immunization and infectious diseases
21. Clinical preventive services

Surveillance and Data Systems
22. Surveillance and data systems

Source: United States Department of Health and Human Services, *Healthy People 2000: Midyear Review and 1995 Revisions* (see reference list), p. iv.

to at least 65 years. Progress toward achieving the objectives is sum-marized each year in the annual publication *Health United States* (e.g., United States Department of Health and Human Services, 1998a), and periodically in such publications as *Healthy People 2000 Review: 1998–1999* (United States Department of Health and Human Services, 1999).

In 1998, a new initiative was undertaken by the Surgeon General of the United States, Dr. David Satcher (United States Department of Health and Human Services, 1998b), to develop a new set of Healthy People Objectives for the year 2010. In his introduction to the "Draft for Public Comment," Dr. Satcher said:

> This next set of national objectives will be distinguished from *Healthy People 2000* by the broadened prevention science base; improved surveillance and data systems; a heightened awareness and demand for preventive health services and quality health care; and changes in demographics, science, technology, and disease spread that will affect the public's health in the 21st century. (p. 1)

Obviously, the general approach to health promotion and disease prevention works, but much remains to be done. There is a still-unfulfilled promise. Among others, the interventions discussed in this book certainly can play a significant role in fulfilling it. It is to be hoped that if and when a comprehensive national health care system, providing a minimum package of services to all residents at little or no cost at the time/point of service (common to all other developed countries), is finally established in the United States, sig-nificant attention to the achievement of the established health pro-motion/disease prevention objectives, as called for in the original Clinton Health Plan of 1993, will be provided for.

VI. THE HP/DP INTERVENTIONS AND THEIR EFFECTIVENESS

Effective interventions for dealing with risk-factors are discussed at length in such works as the *Guide to Clinical Preventive Services*, Second Edition (United States Preventive Services Task Force, 1996); *The Clinician's Handbook of Preventive Services* (Agency for Health

Care Policy and Research, 1998); and the textbooks *Health Promotion and Disease Prevention in Clinical Practice* (Woolf, Jonas, & Lawrence, 1996), *Health Promotion Handbook* (Gorin & Arnold, 1998), and *Maxcy-Rosenau-Last: Public Health and Preventive Medicine* (Wallace, 1998).

To consider the scientific basis of many common health promotive/disease preventive measures, "An Assessment of the Effectiveness of 169 Interventions" used for personal health promotion/disease prevention efforts was carried out by the U.S. Preventive Services Task Force, created by the Office of Disease Prevention and Health Promotion of the U.S. Department of Health and Human Services. Its first report, the *Guide to Clinical Preventive Services*, was published in 1989 (United States Preventive Services Task Force, 1989). As noted, the second edition was published in 1996 (1996).

The Task Force approached the analysis of the health promotive/disease preventive interventions in the manner in which all health services interventions should be analyzed. Among the questions the Task Force asked were: What is the evidence of effectiveness? Is there convincing evidence that the intervention should be made part of the standard package of clinical services? Alternatively, should unproven procedures be allowed, even encouraged, to be widely diffused, as if often the case in the curative medical sector?

While one can strongly support broad recognition of the importance of preventive services and their incorporation into the routine clinical practice, one should also agree with the Task Force that they should be proven to be of benefit before they are broadly offered. Underlining the importance of this point, the Task Force did identify a number of common preventive interventions that are not effective or probably not effective.

VII. THE PERSONAL/COMMUNITY INTERFACE IN HP/DP

Most HP/DP interventions engaged in by clinicians (as contrasted with those engaged in by public health practitioners) concern personal behavior. Therefore, as noted in chapter 1, this book focuses primarily on personal behavior changes as promoters of health. And within the realm of personal behavior, I deal primarily with those change factors that are or can be under a person's control.

This is not to say, however, that dealing with harmful environmental and genetic/familial factors is not also critically important for the prevention of disease and the promotion of health in the population as a whole. As noted in the AJHP definition of Health Promotion quoted at the beginning of this chapter and the work of Dr. Breslow cited in chapters 1 and 5, on balance such interventions are perhaps even more valuable in improving *population* health levels than personal HP/DP measures are. But just as treatment medicine certainly benefits many individuals who receive it, so does personal HP/DP benefit those who undertake it.

As an example of the community/personal HP/DP interface, consider the use of alcohol and nicotine in tobacco by children (the age group in which most use of these drugs starts). An effective primary prevention program will focus primarily on the related environmental factors. These include two of the major causes of the use of these drugs by children: alcohol and tobacco advertising and the ready, relatively cheap, for-the-most-part uncontrolled availability of both substances to children (despite laws prohibiting their sale to underage persons).

However, for *current* smokers and drinkers, quitting is obviously a personal behavior change, much more the purview of the clinician. And, to the extent that individual clinical practitioners, operating in the context of the provider-patient/client interaction, can help people to make health-promoting personal behavior change(s), to that extent can the clinician also contribute to improving the health of the population, as well as helping each individual.

VIII. USING HP/DP INTERVENTIONS

For the clinician, the key to helping people improve their personal health status is effective communication, which we will discuss in some detail in chapter 6. To be an effective communicator in the realm of behavior change, the clinician obviously must have good communication skills, from speaking clearly to presenting HP/DP information in a nonthreatening way. However, all talk and no content makes Jack/Jacqueline a not-very-convincing-or-believable boy or girl. To be able to communicate most effectively, the clinician must also have a thorough understanding of the nature of the subject about which she or he is communicating, in this case HP/DP.

Since HP/DP interventions are much talked about but not so widely practiced in our health care delivery system, patients/clients will often not have a basic familiarity with their processes. (In contrast, they often are familiar with the basic processes of disease management.) Therefore, in the view of this book, to be maximally effective health care professionals should be able to assist their patients/clients in learning that set of central HP/DP Concepts (as noted in the formulation presented in this book there are 10) that will be helpful to them. It is to an examination of these Concepts that we now turn.

REFERENCES

AHCPR: Agency for Health Care Policy and Research (1998). *Clinician's handbook of preventive services.* Washington, DC: U.S. Dept. of Health and Human Services, Office of Public Health and Science.

Breslow, L. (1996). Social Ecological Strategies for Promoting Healthy Lifestyles. *American Journal of Health Promotion, 10,* 253.

Downie, R. S., Tannahill, C., & Tannahill, A. (1996). *Health promotion: Models and values.* New York: Oxford University Press.

Gorin, S. S., & Arnold, J. (1998). *Health Promotion Handbook.* St. Louis, MO: Mosby.

Hoyert, D. L., Kochanek, K. D., & Murphy, S. L. (1999, June 30). Deaths: Final Date for 1997. *National Vital Statistics Reports, 47.*

Jonas, S. (1998). *An Introduction to the U.S. Health Care System* (4th ed.). New York: Springer Publishing.

McGinniss, J. M. (1990). Prevention in 1989: The State of the Nation. *American Journal of Preventive Medicine, 6,* 1–5.

McGinniss, J. M., & Foege, W. H. (1993). Actual Causes of Death in the United States. *Journal of the American Medical Association, 270,* 2207–2212.

McKeown, T. (1976). *The role of medicine: Dream, mirage, or nemesis.* London: The Nuffield Provincial Hospitals Trust.

McKeown, T. (1997). Determinants of Health. In Lee, P. R. & Estes, C. L. (Eds.), *The nation's health* (5th ed.). Boston, MA: Jones and Bartlett.

(1997). State- and Sex-Specific Prevalence of Selected Characteristics—Behavioral Risk Factor Surveillance System, 1994 and 1995. *Morbidity and Mortality Weekly Report, 46*.

(1999a). Ten Great Public Health Achievements—United States, 1900–1999. *Morbidity and Mortality Weekly Report, 48*, 241–243.

(1999b). Decline in Deaths Heart Disease and Stroke—United States, 1900–1999, *Morbidity and Mortality Weekly Report, 48*, 649–656.

O'Donnell, M. P. (1989). Definition of Health Promotion: Part III: Expanding the Definition. *American Journal of Health Promotion, 3*, 5.

Sigerist, H. (1941). *Medicine and human welfare.* New Haven, CT: Yale University Press.

Tannahill, A. (1985). What is health promotion? *Health Education Journal, 44*, 167–168.

USDHEW: US Department of Health, Education, and Welfare. (1979). *Healthy people: The surgeon general's report on health promotion and disease prevention.* Washington, DC: Author. (DHEW [PHS] Pub. No. 79-55071).

U.S. Department of Health and Human Services. (1991). *Healthy People 2000: National Health Promotion and Disease Prevention Objectives,* Washington, DC: US Public Health Service. (DHHS Pub. No. [PHS] 91-50213).

U.S. Dept. of Health and Human Services. (1995). *Healthy People 2000: Mid-Course Review and 1995 Revisions.* Washington, DC: U.S. Public Health Service.

U.S. Department of Health and Human Services. (1998a). *Health, United States, 1998, With Socioeconomic Status and Health Chartbook.* Hyattsville, MD: National Center for Health Statistics. (DHHS Pub. No. [PHS] 98-1232).

U.S. Department of Health and Human Services. (1998b). *Healthy People 2010 Objectives: Draft for Public Comment.* Washington, DC: Office of Public Health and Science.

U.S. Department of Health and Human Services. (1999). *Healthy People 2000 Review 1998–99.* Hyattsville, MD: Centers for Disease Control and Prevention. (DHHS Pub. No. [PHS] 99-1256).

United States Preventive Services Task Force. (1989). *Guide to clinical preventive services.* Baltimore, MD: Williams and Wilkins.

United States Preventive Services Task Force. (1996). *Guide to clinical preventive services* (2nd ed.). Baltimore, MD: Williams and Wilkins.

Wallace, W. B. (1998). *Maxcy-Rosenau-Last: Public health and preventive medicine* (14th ed.). Norwalk, CT: Appleton & Lange.

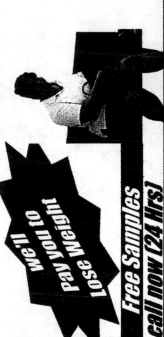

Weinerman, E. R. (1971). Research on Comparative Health Service Systems. *Medical Care, 9,* 272.

Woolf, S. H., Jonas, S., & Lawrence, R. (Eds.). (1996). *Health promotion and disease prevention in clinical practice.* Baltimore, MD: Williams and Wilkins.

Wynder, E., & Kristein, M. (1977). Suppose We Died Young, Late in Life? *Journal of the American Medical Association, 238,* 1507.

THE TEN CONTRAL CONCEPTS

Chapter 4

THE SUBSTANTIVE CENTRAL CONCEPTS: Numbers I–VII

INTRODUCTION

Each of the Ten Central Concepts of Health Promotion/Disease Prevention (HP/DP) embodies an idea the use of which is intended to improve the chances of success in a clinical intervention focussed on health and wellness. As noted in chapter 1, the Ten Central Concepts fall into two groups. The first seven are the primarily *substantive* common denominators of virtually all personal HP/DP activities/interventions. The three Concepts that primarily concern the *process* of individual behavior change comprise the second group.

The primarily substantive Concepts concern *what* health, wellness, and health promotion are and how they are characterized, both conceptually and as used in the clinical setting. The Concepts focussed primarily on the process of individual behavior change deal with *how* one goes about becoming and being both healthy and well, on the personal level. Of course, each Concept has elements of both substance and process, but they are grouped according to which of these two defining characteristics is the most prominent in each. The seven substantive Concepts are discussed in this chapter, the three that concern process in the next one.

The seven substantive Concepts are:

  I.   Health is a state of being; wellness is a process of being.
  II. Health status is determined by a broad range of factors.
  III. Health has a natural history.
  IV. Central to the wellness process is a wide array of HP/DP interventions.
  V.   Success in certain behavior change endeavors is relative.
  VI. Risks to health can be reduced; in few instances is there certainty of outcome.
  VII. Achieving balance is the essence of healthy living and wellness.

CONCEPT I. HEALTH IS A STATE OF BEING; WELLNESS IS A PROCESS OF BEING

As illustrated in chapter 2, the term "health" has been defined in many ways. The definitions presented there range from the simple (some would say simplistic) "the absence of disease," to the complex (see the next paragraph). Common to most of these definitions is the idea that the terms "health" and "healthy" in one way or another describe an individual's state of being at a given time. Also common to most definitions of health is the underlying assumption that at a given time a person's level of health, their "healthiness" if you will, can be measured and evaluated. The results of the variety of measurements and evaluative processes that can be used to carry out that task together describe a person's state of being, in terms of health.

We can see that this is so upon revisiting the consolidated definition of health offered in chapter 2 (p. 15):

> *Health* is a positive, balanced, state of being characterized by the best achievable physical, psychological, emotional, social, spiritual and intellectual levels of functioning at a given time, the absence of disease or the optimal management of chronic disease, and the control of both internal and external risk factors for both diseases and negative health conditions.

The measures that can be used to evaluate the health and health status of an individual range from the simple question "how do you feel?" to various tests of physical and mental functioning. Among these latter measures are: medical/health history taking; screening (for clinically inapparent disease); diagnostic laboratory tests, imaging, and other procedures (for clinically apparent disease); and the completion by the individual of various questionnaires designed to measure, for example, mental status or occupational preference/aptitude.

The outcomes of these measures and measurements can be expressed in words, numbers, or images. They can then be compared with known normal, "healthy" ranges, based on findings in population groups. Criteria have been developed for the outcomes of virtually all available measurements. They can be expressed as indicating, for example: "healthy, somewhat healthy, has a way to go, unhealthy;" "within/not-within the normal/healthy range found in the population tested," "illustrating the presence of an unhealthy condition."

Thus, at any given time the health status of an individual can be characterized in objective terms (e.g., using numbers; seeing the presence/absence of an abnormal mass on diagnostic imaging), or in subjective ones that nevertheless are reproducible: "I feel/do not feel fine."

Of course, as previously noted, even in the healthiest of people health status varies over time. How it varies, and what one does to influence that variation and its direction (toward/away from a healthy *state of being*) determines whether one is engaged in the *process* of "wellness." Recall Dr. Dunn's definition of "high level wellness" (Dunn, 1961/1977):

> an integrated method of functioning which is oriented toward maximizing the potential of which the individual is capable. It requires that the individual maintain a continuum of balance and purposeful direction within the environment where he is functioning. (p. 4)

We can then say that the more well one is, the more oriented toward achieving and maintaining a state of health in the broadest sense of the term one is at any given time throughout the course of one's life. Thus the level of wellness, that is how engaged one is in the process of striving towards health, can be measured, just as health status can be measured. But once again, the latter is a measure of *something existing at a given time*, while the former is a measure of *something going on over time*. Another way of looking at the nature of health and wellness is that at any given time, an individual's state of health represents an intermediate outcome in the life-long process of wellness.

CONCEPT II. HEALTH STATUS IS DETERMINED BY A BROAD RANGE OF FACTORS

As discussed in chapters 2 and 3, a person's state of health is influenced/determined by a broad range of factors. Environmental and genetic ones are critically important, as noted. For example, for the working population the structure and functioning of the workplace is key, as is, for students, the structure and functioning of the academic setting. As noted in chapter 2, in his recent work Don Ardell has emphasized the major role that the *political/economic* environment in which one lives plays in determining one's health level and degree of wellness (Ardell, 1999).

Nevertheless, as you, dear reader, know by now, this book focuses primarily on the individual/personal factors determining a person's health status at any given time *that are or can be under the person's control*, and what he or she may be able to do about them over time, in particular with the help of a clinician. Comprising this group is what can be termed the "Big Ten Personal Factors of Health." (This list has much in common with the health promotion section of the *Healthy People 2000* "Priority Areas" (*see* Table 3.1.) They are:

1. Physical activity status.
2. Weight and body fat proportion.
3. Dietary composition.
4. Use or nonuse of tobacco products.
5. Use or nonuse, on a nonprescription basis, of mood-altering drugs* legally requiring prescription by a physician, dentist, or designee.
6. Use or nonuse of alcohol and the other recreational mood-altering drugs*.

---

* A drug is any substance other than food that by its chemical nature affects the structure or function of the living organism (Jonas, 1997, p. 775). A "mood-

7. How internal and external stressors are managed.
8. Use (or not) of safe sexual practices.
9. How personal safety at home, in private and public transport, and at the workplace is protected.
10. Immune status.

As is well known, in dealing with the Big Ten Personal Factors of Health, for an individual the following program would be optimal:

• Engaging in a suitable regular exercise program.
• Having a body weight and fat proportion that reasonably corresponds to normal for one's age, sex, and height.
• Eating a reasonably balanced diet containing a moderate level of fat.
• Using neither tobacco products nor prescription mood-altering drugs on a nonprescription basis.
• Using alcohol or any of the other recreational mood-altering drugs in moderation, if at all.
• Handling stress productively.
• Practicing safe sex.
• Protecting personal safety (without becoming obsessive about it).
• Maintaining an up-to-date, age-appropriate immune status.

In helping patients and clients to develop their own "Big Ten" program, there is a common problem traditionally trained clinicians face when dealing with health rather than disease. Not everyone can do everything they could do. In a given patient/client presenting with one factor of the Big Ten that stands out as not being under reasonable control, there is often the tendency to focus on that one factor to the exclusion of others.

Thus with the overweight person *the* issue becomes their weight and what they might be able to do to reduce it. With the cigarette smoker *the* issue becomes quitting. With the highly nervous, tense person *the* issue becomes effective stress management. But at any

---

altering drug" is one that in one way or another affects one's state of mind and feelings. A "recreational mood-altering drug" is one that is ingested, inhaled, or injected for the primary purpose of providing diversion, relaxation, heightened sensation, or other enjoyment and pleasure by changing the user's state of mind.

given time, one's overall health status is not determined by just one of the Big Ten Factors of Health. It is determined by all of them (as well as many others beyond the direct control of any individual) and by the interplay among them.

Take overweight as an example. Losing weight is probably the single most difficult personal health-promoting activity anyone can undertake. The long-term success rate in weight loss is variously reported as between 5% and 10% (Jonas & Konner, 1997, p. 11). (In contrast, about 50% of those who attempt to quit smoking are ultimately successful [Schmitz, Schneider, & Jarvik, 1997, p. 276].) This is the situation in the United States, in the context of an obesity epidemic (Jonas & Konner, 1997, p. 10; Wickelgren, 1998) and the environment that feeds it (Hill & Peters, 1998). (The latter includes a much-more-than-ample food supply [for most, although sadly not all, Americans], easy availability of high-fat foods, and large portion sizes at most restaurants.) There is also a common mode of weight-loss dieting, used especially by women, that alters metabolism and makes it doubly difficult to lose weight (Jonas, 1993).

At the same time, there is a media-propelled popular culture that stresses thinness as the beauty ideal, especially for women. Many women thus get caught up in the no-win cycle of weight gain/weight loss, in the context of the constant social pressure to lose (Jonas & Konner, 1997, p. 12). Part of this social pressure is the constant emphasis not only on the cosmetic aspects of overweight, but on the negative health aspects of it as well (Polivy, 1999). At times, women in particular can develop a monomaniacal focus on weight loss, despite the fact that it is so difficult to achieve.

However, if we recognize the spectrum of factors that influence health, even just those that are potentially under a person's control, we can see that it is possible for the overweight person to be otherwise healthy (Jonas & Konner, 1997; Miller, 1997). And if one simply cannot lose weight no matter how hard one tries, or if one does not *want* to lose weight for one reason or another, one neither has to feel that one is forever condemned to a life of bad health, nor should one be objectively considered totally unhealthy, just because one factor is not where it should be.

For the overweight person can exercise regularly (even if one doesn't lose weight), eat a balanced diet (even if one doesn't lose weight), not use tobacco products or any of the mood-altering drugs other than alcohol in moderation, for the most part effectively manage stress, promote (but not to excess) personal safety, practice safe sex, and keep immune status up-to-date. And overweight or not, such a person could indeed be considered to be, on balance, in good health, (Jonas & Konner, 1997).

Indeed, Steven Blair and colleagues of the Aerobics Institute in Dallas, Texas found that in two groups of men, one overweight but exercising, the other normal weight, but not exercising, it was the former that had the better long-term health outcomes (Blair, et al., 1996; Lee, Blair, & Jackson, 1999). It is obvious that for the clinician concerned with health and wellness this perspective of balance should be kept very much in mind (see also Concept VII).

CONCEPT III: HEALTH HAS A NATURAL HISTORY

For any given individual, whatever that person's health, that "positive, balanced, state of being," the product of the interaction of all those factors that influence it at any given time, varies over time. And what one is realistically *capable* of doing for oneself in terms of one's own health, that is the extent to which one can stay on the wellness pathway, also varies over time.

The spectrum of personal health factors described in Concept II, existing and measurable at any given time, can be characterized as the "horizontal" aspect of health. The changes over time in both the Big Ten Factors and overall health status can be considered the "vertical" aspect of health. Together, these observations provide the essence of the Concept that health has a natural history, just as disease does.

In the course of their studies, most health professional students become familiar with what is called "the natural history of disease." Thus we learn that heart disease begins with the first deposition of a piece of plaque in the wall of a coronary artery. In some persons over time, through a variety of stages plaque accumulates until the coronary artery becomes blocked. Beyond that site, cardiac muscle dies, leading in many cases to the occurrence of what is called a "heart attack." A similar scenario could be written for the development of cancer, diabetes, cirrhosis of the liver, and so on.

In health by the same token, looking at the Big Ten Factors we can see that the expression of each one can and does change over time in each person as well. Body weight can and often does go up and down. One's activity status changes. One is a smoker and then one quits. And so forth. What also changes is one's *interest* in doing anything about any of the Factors that may be in a negative state at a given time, and the *ability* to make such a change if the interest is there. Certainly, the *capability* to successfully make a positive behavior change takes *both* interest and ability.

Age is obviously a critical variable in whether one has the capability of making health-promoting change(s) at any given time. In many people, body weight increases with age, naturally. If one has never been physically active, the older one gets the more difficult it is to become so, just from the mechanical point of view. On the other hand, growing older many people become calmer as they arrive at a more mature perspective on life and its vicissitudes. For some that makes it easier to deal productively with external stressors.

But at different times in one's life positive or negative changes in one or more of the Big Ten can occur with utter unpredictability. Sometimes an individual will know when he or she is ready to make a positive, health-promoting behavior change and understand why the change in attitude occurred at that time. At other times, the "learning moment" occurs with no rational explanation for "why then?" not 6 months earlier or 6 years later.

Take the example of a 43-year-old man who has never been athletic, who has never been in any kind of "shape" in his life. For several years he has been thinking about taking up running to improve his health and fitness, but other than buying several books on the subject, he has done nothing about it. One October Tuesday morning, at an Annual Meeting of the American Public Health Association being held in Detroit, Michigan, he is trudging up a one-flight ramp in Cobo Hall to give a talk on political lobbying. Reaching the top of the ramp, as usual when engaging in a like activity, he is out of breath. As not usual for him, however, this time he says to himself: "I just don't like being this way. When I get home I'm going to begin running, doing the American College of Sports Medicine recommended 20 minutes, three times per week. I know I'm going to hate it, but I've just got to do it."

And so, when he gets home he starts a walk/run program with the goal of being able to run for 20 minutes without stopping. It takes him a month to achieve that goal. But along the way, he finds that not only doesn't he hate it; actually he likes it. Three years later, he finishes his first triathlon*, and 17 years after that he finishes his 100th multisport event. For this previous nonathlete, regular exercise and sport have become a major part of his life. He discovered that he could do things he had never even thought about, much less contemplated undertaking. He also reaped a harvest of mental benefits that were even more important to him than the physical ones.

Why did the change happen when it happened? Who knows. But the "why/when" is really unimportant. That it happened is. In the natural history of this man's health, the event of his becoming a regular exerciser occurred when he was 43 years old. It might have happened earlier, and it might have happened later, but it did happen. To be an effective promoter of health, the clinician must understand this phenomenon.

We must be patient with our patients and clients, and we must be patient with ourselves in dealing with them. Just because we think that a patient should do thus and such, now, or that a client thinks that the client should do thus and such, then, doesn't mean that at that particular time that person is truly ready to make, and is capable of making, that particular change.

Neither does it mean that that person will not be ready to make, and be capable of making, that particular change 6 months or a year down the road. One must enable one's patients/clients to develop this perspective and maintain their optimism. Just easing off on the "must," "should," "right now" ethic can be marvelously liberating, and possibly facilitating for the change process in the future. Understanding, recognizing, and using this Concept are how the two components of Concept I—health is a state of being and wellness is a process of being—are integrated in the care of our patients and clients.

---

* A triathlon is a multisport race, usually including swimming, cycling, and running, in which the segments (one of each sport) are done consecutively. The other common multisport race is the duathlon, a three segment/two sport (run-bike-run) event.

CONCEPT IV. CENTRAL TO THE WELLNESS PROCESS IS A WIDE ARRAY OF HP/DP INTERVENTIONS

As noted in chapter 1, that set of activities/interventions known as Health Promotion establishes the programmatic base for persons engaging in the wellness process over the course of their lifetimes. As noted in chapter 2, the following is a useful definition of health promotion (developed for the *American Journal of Health Promotion* (O'Donnell, 1989):

> Health promotion is the science and art of helping people change their lifestyle to move toward a state of optimal health. Optimal health is defined as a balance of physical, emotional, social, spiritual and intellectual health. Life-style change can be facilitated through a combination of efforts to enhance awareness, change behavior and create environments that support good health practices. Of the three, supportive environments will probably have the greatest impact in producing lasting change.

The movement toward "a state of optimal health" describes the lifetime process of wellness, as we have seen. There is obviously an array of interventions/activities that is part of the process (see also Concept II). That array ranges from "pure" prevention (immunization) to improving one's spiritual well-being through meditation. Further, because such health promoting activities as regular exercise can improve one's spiritual health too, there is obviously a seamless web among and between the various components of the spectrum. Each is supportive of the other. Thus there are no dichotomies between and among prevention, health promotion, and wellness advocacy.

As noted in Concept II, paralleling the Big Ten controllable personal health factors is a Big Ten Set of Health Promoting Personal Behaviors/Activities:

1. Exercising regularly.
2. Managing one's weight.
3. Eating a healthy diet.
4. Not smoking or otherwise using tobacco products.
5. Not using the prescription mood-altering drugs on a nonprescription basis.

6. Safe use of the recreational mood-altering drugs such as alcohol or, if one must use them, any of the illicits.
7. Managing one's internal and external stressors effectively.
8. Using safe sexual practices.
9. Protecting personal safety at home, in the car, and at the workplace.
10. Maintaining immune status at the effective level.

Consistent with the definition of "optimal health" is that each one of the Big Ten Set can, and often does, have an impact on one or more of the emotional, social, spiritual, and intellectual aspects of health as well as on the physical ones. For example, while becoming a regular exerciser certainly improves one's physical health, in most cases it also helps clients to feel better and feel better about themselves. Exercising regularly may also help one to make new friends, develop new understandings of the meaning of life, and improve one's rational thought processes.

In working with patients and clients, clinicians need to make judgments and help patients to set priorities for incorporating one or more of the Big Ten Set of activities into their own lives at any one time. One approach to this task is to divide the Big Ten into two groups: a "mandatory minimum" of healthy behaviors for achieving a healthy state, and a second set, recommended, but not absolutely required at any given point in time.

The first group includes not smoking, a minimal level of healthy eating, nonuse of the prescription recreational mood-altering drugs on a nonprescription basis, nonabuse of the other recreational mood-altering drugs, the practice of safe sex, and a healthy immunization status. The second, then, includes regular exercise, weight approaching the recommended mean, effective stress management, and attention to personal safety issues.

CONCEPT V. SUCCESS IN CERTAIN BEHAVIOR CHANGE ENDEAVORS IS RELATIVE

"Success" in working with the Big Ten health promotion/disease prevention interventions means making positive lifestyle changes to improve one's health, to feel better, and feel better about oneself.

As we have noted, there are certain absolutes for leading a healthy life, such as not smoking cigarettes, not abusing alcoholic beverages, practicing safe sex. However, it is very important to understand that while for those behaviors "improving one's health" and "feeling better" require an absolute outcome, in others, like regular exercise and weight loss, they do not.

At any one time, for the latter "health improvement" can and does have different meanings for different people. And over time, as expressed in Concept III, "health has a natural history," they can and do have different meanings for the same person. What defines "success" in these realms for one person does not necessarily do it for another. By the same token, what defines "success" for a person at one time in his or her life is not necessarily what does it at another time. Thus for health-related behaviors other than those that require absolute outcomes, in goal setting for behavior change (see the next chapter) it is vitally important that the goals set are reasonably achievable for the person setting them.

Take regular exercise. What constitutes "success" for a morbidly obese person is quite different from what constitutes it for a person of normal weight. For example, a 400-pound man starting an exercise program might require 67 minutes to walk a mile. A year later, and 100 pounds lighter, he might be walking a mile in 30 minutes, and a year after that, another 50 pounds lighter, he might be walking a mile in 17 minutes. At each level *he* has achieved "success," in terms relative to what he was reasonably capable of achieving. Now, for a person of normal weight becoming a regular exerciser, being able to walk a mile in 67 or even 30 minutes would not ordinarily be considered "successful." But for our formerly morbidly obese man, it is.

At a different level, after 6 months of training a formerly nonathletic woman of normal weight may well be comfortably covering 20 road miles on her bicycle in an hour and a half. By the end of the following season she may have ridden her first "century" (100 miles) in 10 hours (a modest pace for that distance), including a couple of stops for refreshment and rest. For her, that's "success." Our morbidly obese man could do none of this, but given from whence he started he should be considered no less "successful."

And then there is our 43-year-old male with no background in running, cycling, or swimming. Within 3 years of starting to run 20 minutes, three times per week, he has become a triathlete, finishing short-course races on a regular basis, coming in at the back-of-the-pack, but feeling both happy and healthy. For him, propelled by a growing love for this new-found leisure-time pursuit, this is "success." Our century rider could do none of this—no interest, and anyway she can't swim. But she should be considered no less "successful" either. No absolutes; only what's right for and what can/will work for the given individual.

CONCEPT VI. RISKS TO HEALTH CAN BE REDUCED; IN FEW INSTANCES IS THERE CERTAINTY OF OUTCOME

Recall that a risk factor is some environmental element, personal habit, or condition of living that increases the likelihood of developing a particular disease or negative health condition at some time in the future. In medicine, we tend to be taught certainty: plaque causes heart attacks; the right pill will cure the disease it is aimed at; the right surgical procedure will repair the physical defect it has been designed to mend. But in most cases HP/DP interventions are about risk and its reduction.

If one stops smoking cigarettes, or has never started in the first place, we cannot say that one will definitely not develop chronic obstructive pulmonary disease or get lung cancer. Sadly, smoker's lung cancer does occasionally occur in nonsmokers. We can say only that the *risk* of contracting either will be significantly reduced. If one exercises regularly, we cannot say that one will never have a heart attack, only that the *risk* of having one will be significantly reduced. If one maintains a reasonably normal weight, we cannot say that one will never contract diabetes or develop hypertension, only that the *risk* of doing so will be significantly reduced. (On the other hand, proper immunization against a given set of viral diseases virtually does guarantee that one will never contract them.)

Thus, with the exception of immunization, in HP/DP the only guarantee accompanying risk factor reduction/elimination is that the *likelihood* of getting the related disease or negative health condition will be diminished. This is an important concept to convey to patients and clients. Of course, that living a healthy life, being on the wellness pathway, confers many other benefits besides disease prevention can help to sweeten that message.

CONCEPT VII: BALANCE IS THE DYNAMIC GOAL OF HEALTHY LIVING

As Donald and Nancy Loving Tubesing have pointed out, the essence of healthy living is achieving balance in one's life (1991): "taking care of ourselves, investing in meaningful work, and reaching out to others" (p. 6). And recall the definition of health adopted for this book:

Health is a positive, balanced, state of being characterized by the best achievable physical, psychological, emotional, social, spiritual and intellectual levels of functioning at a given time, the absence of disease or the optimal management of chronic disease, and the control of both internal and external risk factors for both diseases and negative health conditions.

How can we help our patients and clients to achieve balance as they move along the wellness pathway? First of all, most people who do make significant changes in their lives almost invariably do so slowly, one step at a time. Many are guided by the following aphorism:

Gradual change leads to permanent changes.

That is, if one makes change slowly, one is much more likely to reach one's goal in the end and maintain it. For example, in weight loss aiming to lose 1 to 2 pounds per week instead of 10 pounds in seven days, or in going to a low-fat diet and planning to convert a total of five meat meals per week to chicken/fish/vegetable meals, doing so by eliminating one meat meal per week rather than trying to do it all at once. Doing it this way will definitely help one achieve balance in one's life.

A second helpful aphorism is:

Explore your limits; recognize your limitations.

In exercise and athletics this means, for example, if one is naturally slow, recognizing that as a limitation, accepting it, working with it. But then one is released to begin exploring one's limits in, say, how far one can go. Thus, once having embarked on the journey of regular exercise, the couch potato can become a marathoner or a triathlete. With a weight-training program a "97 pounds weakling" can develop a nicely formed physique with a significant increase in strength. An uncoordinated, large-size person can become an aerobic dance queen.

However, it is very important to note that while the couch potato may become a marathoner, she may very well be one for whom the ultimate achievement is to finish not in under 3 hours but in under 5. That's keeping things in balance. For the triathlete, the ultimate achievement may not ever be finishing first in his age group in any race, but in completing an ironman-distance triathlon (2.4-mile swim, 112-mile bike, 26.2 mile run) in under the 17-hour time limit. That's keeping things in balance. The "97-pound weakling" may become strong, but on his own terms, such as, being able to bench press 120 pounds, not 275 pounds. And "well-formed" for this man will mean reducing his body-fat proportion to 17% from 25%, not to the 4% of a professional body-builder. That's keeping things in balance.

For our aerobic dancer, success may well mean that she is happy to regularly attend a 1-hour class three times per week, doing the whole routine comfortably at the instructor's pace, having gone from 40% overweight for her age, height, and body frame-size to 20% overweight. For her, it will *not* mean that she becomes a size 6, with the ability to lead five classes a day, 6 days per week. That's keeping things in balance, too.

Finally, to achieve balance, a third aphorism, this time a self-explanatory one, may be found useful:

You can always get better; you can never be perfect. That being so, with certain exceptions,* perfectioni*sm* in health promotion/

---

* Those exceptions are, as noted previously: not using tobacco products; not abusing alcohol or any of the other recreational mood-altering drugs; not using prescription psychoactive drugs on a nonprescription basis; always practicing safe sex; and maintaining a healthy immune status.

disease prevention is a destructive, not a constructive, state of mind.

And so, we are now ready to move on to a consideration of how we help our patients and clients to get where they want to go. We thus turn to the Process Concepts.

REFERENCES

Ardell, D. B. (1999, Summer). What is Wellness. *Ardell Wellness Report, 53,* 1.

Blair, S., et al. (1996). Influences of Cardiorespiratory Fitness and Other Precursors on Cardiovascular Disease and All-Cause Mortality in Men and Women. *Journal of the American Medical Association, 276,* 205–210.

Dunn, H. L. (1961/1977). *High-level wellness.* Thorofare, NJ: Charles B. Slack.

Hill, J. O., & Peters, J. C. (1998). Environmental Contributions to the Obesity Epidemic. *Science, 280,* 1371.

Jonas, S. (1993). *Take control of your weight.* Yonkers, NY: Consumers Reports Books.

Jonas, S. (1997). Public Health Approaches. In J. H. Lowinson, et al. (Eds.), *Substance abuse: A comprehensive textbook.* Baltimore, MD: Williams & Wilkins.

Jonas, S., & Konner, L. (1997). *Just the weigh you are: How to be fit and healthy, whatever your size.* Boston, MA: Chapters/Houghton Mifflin.

Lee, C. D., Blair, C. N., & Jackson, A. S. (1999). Cardiorespiratory fitness, body composition, and all-cause and cardiovascular disease mortality in men. *American Journal of Clinical Nutrition, 69,* 373–380.

Miller, W. C. (1997). *Negotiated peace.* Needham Heights, MA: Allyn & Bacon.

O'Donnell, M. P. (1989). Definition of Health Promotion: Part III: Expanding the Definition. *American Journal of Health Promotion, 3,* 5.

Polivy, J. (1999). The Mythology of Dieting. *Healthy Weight Journal, 13,* 1.

Schmitz, J. M., Schneider, N. G., & Jarvik, M. E. (1997). Nicotine. In *Substance abuse: A comprehensive textbook.* 3rd ed., J. H. Lowinson, P. Ruiz, R. B. Millman, & J. B. Langrod (Eds.) Baltimore, MD: Williams & Wilkins.

Tubesing, D. A., & Tubesing, N. L. (1991). *Seeking your healthy balance: A do-it-yourself guide to whole person well-being*. Duluth, MN: Whole Person Associates.

Wickelgren, I. (1998). Obesity: How Big a Problem? *Science, 280*, 1364.

THE PROCESS CENTRAL CONCEPTS: Numbers VIII–X

INTRODUCTION

This chapter focusses on the processes of personal lifestyle/behavior change common to the Big Ten set of personal health promoting interventions discussed in the previous chapter. It provides information about how clinicians can help patients learn to use these Concepts in making changes in the way they live their lives.

There are only three Central Concepts of Health Promotion/Disease Prevention (HP/DP) concerned primarily with process. They represent a single common pathway that will be followed by patients and clients in making any one of the behavior changes common to the Big Ten, regardless of the nature of the change: becoming a regular exerciser, losing weight, stopping smoking, and so forth. Each element is essential and essentially the same if any contemplated behavior change is to be successfuly made.

CONCEPT VIII: THERE IS A COMMON PATHWAY TO SUCCESS FOR MOST PERSONAL BEHAVIOR CHANGE EFFORTS

A model of the psychological change process that underlies virtually all positive health-related lifestyle/behavior changes was originally developed by Prochaska and DiClemente (1982). Often referred to as the "Stages of Change" model, it is widely used. In the early 1990s, the work was updated (Prochaska, 1993; Prochaska, DiClemente, & Norcross, 1992; Prochaska, Norcross, & DiClemente, 1992; Prochaska & Velicer, 1997; Velicer & Prochaska, 1997). This description and analysis of the change process is very helpful in understanding how lifestyle/personal behavior can be successfully altered (and also in understanding why the process sometimes fails).

In their revision of the original model, Prochaska, DiClemente, and Norcross (1992) identify what they call "The Six Stages of Change"

- Precontemplation
- Contemplation
- Preparation
- Action
- Maintenance
- Termination

As Prochaska (1993) pointed out:

In this stage approach to change, taking direct action to change one's behavior is only one of six stages. What people do in the stages preceding action and what they do in the stages following action are at least as important as the action they take. (p. 249)

It is very important to understand that in most people the process of mobilizing motivation and then engaging in behavioral change does not take place overnight (think of the Natural History of Health). In fact, programs that focus solely on the behaviors, and not on attending to the motivational process that underlies behavioral change as well, are more likely than not to lead to failure (Prochaska, 1993). And so, the Stages.

1. PRECONTEMPLATION

In this stage the decision or determination that there is a problem requiring some solution, taking some action, making a change, has not yet been made. There is no intent to take any action within the upcoming 6 months. The calculation has been made that the benefits of inaction are at least as great, if not greater, than the benefits of taking action. There may be an unawareness, or at least not a full awareness, of the potential benefits of making a change, or there may be a demoralization arising from past unsuccessful attempts at change. Thus, there is an acceptance of the present state of being, either happily or unhappily.

2. CONTEMPLATION

In this stage a measure of self-awareness makes its appearance. There is a recognition that a behavior such as living a sedentary lifestyle constitutes a health-related problem. There is an assessment of just what effect current behavior is having on the person. The individual begins to look at different aspects of change. In this stage, a serious intent to take action within the next 6 months or so is established, but no action is taken just yet. There is an awareness of the advantages of making change, and at least part of the mind is in favor of doing it. But at the same time there is still a concern with the cons of change-making (that is, *ambivalence* is present; see also below under "Mobilizing motivation"). A part of the mind may be convinced that success will be difficult, if not impossible, to achieve.

As Miller and Rollnick (1991) said about ambivalence:

> Once some awareness of the problem arises, the person enters a period characterized by *ambivalence*: the "contemplation" stage. The contemplator *both* considers change and rejects it [emphasis added]. (p. 16)

Some people can remain in the contemplation stage for quite some time, even though upon originally entering it they fully intended to make a change within 6 months or so. Distinguishing those who will be able to proceed to the next stage from those who will not is the ability of the former to begin seeing oneself as a person who behaves differently than they do in present time.

3. PREPARATION

In this stage, serious planning to engage in behavior change within the next month is undertaken. Upon entering this stage, one's "motivation has been mobilized." That is, the link between thought and action (see Concept IX) that will get the change process started has been activated. The person has, in the common parlance, "become motivated." Ambivalent feelings and doubts that success can in fact be achieved have been overcome. There has been a conscious choice to engage in a new set of behaviors, and the belief that positive change will indeed be possible has been established. Assessment/self-assessment has been carried out, goals have been set, and a program, formal or informal, for making the desired behavior change has been adopted.

4. ACTION

The next step of the change process is taking the action itself. The chosen program is implemented. In many cases, such as becoming a regular exerciser or a healthy eater, the dictum to be carefully followed is "gradual change leads to permanent changes" (see the previous chapter). In some cases, however, such as those of certain people attempting to quit cigarette smoking, and virtually all who are intending to stop abusing alcohol, the change is made suddenly, "cold turkey" in common parlance.

5. MAINTENANCE

"Maintenance" is the next step on the way to full realization of the desired lifestyle change. It is a way station that will lead either to permanent incorporation of the new behavior into one's life or to a full or partial withdrawal from it. According to the Prochaska and DiClemente model there are three different possible "next steps" after the Maintenance stage: "Lapse," "Relapse," and "Termination." (In this book we refer to "Termination" as "Permanent Maintenance.")

A. LAPSE

Lapse is a temporary abandonment of the positive behavior followed by a quick return to it. Lapse does not produce any *significant* alteration in progress toward established goals or, having achieved them, any significant modification in, say, fitness or body configuration. In fact, in certain endeavors, such as a program of regular exercise, it happens that it is a good idea to voluntarily come to a full stop for 2 to 4 weeks at least annually, just to give both body and mind a rest. (The pauses should not last *too* long, however, lest the person experience a significant decline in fitness level or significant muscular pain upon returning to the activity.)

The key word above is *significant*. For example, for the weight loser on the way toward a goal of a 30-pound weight loss in 6 months, regaining a pound or two after having lost 10 over a month or two, is not significant. That happens to most weight losers. Also, once 30 or 40 pounds are lost, a lapse into some old-style eating followed by a 5-pound regain, but stopping there and returning to the new healthy eating pattern, constitutes nothing to worry about. Thus lapse is just fine, can be fun for a limited time, and is perfectly normal. Worrisome is what is called relapse.

B. RELAPSE

Relapse is abandonment of the positive behaviors that have produced the desired outcomes, to the extent that those outcomes disappear. For example, the program of regular exercise is given up indefinitely. The good feelings, changes in body shape, and increased strength and endurance gained from doing it vanish. To reverse relapse requires first figuring out what happened, why the relapse occurred. Then it requires going back to the preparation stage and recommencing the change process.

It is important to understand that just as being sedentary or over-weight or a smoker of cigarettes is not a sign of moral failure or sin-fulness, neither is relapsing. It just means one of the following:

- There was not a true readiness the first time around; that is, the person's motivation was not effectively mobilized.
- The goals set were unrealistic.
- A goal was simply unachievable, objectively (as, for example, is the case for certain overweight persons in whom for certain physiological and/or psychological reasons significant per-manent weight loss is virtually impossible to achieve regard-less of what they do [Heatherton & Tickle, 1999; Polivy, 1999]).
- That one or more objective circumstances, external or internal, have changed in one way or another.

If relapse occurs, it is important that the natural disappointment accompanying it is not allowed to turn to permanent discourage-ment or demoralization. There are often very good reasons for such an occurrence. It happens to many people, and not by any stretch of the imagination does it necessarily mean that they will not even-tually achieve Permanent Maintenance.

6. PERMANENT MAINTENANCE

Permanent Maintenance ("Termination" in the Prochaska and DiClemente terminology) means that the person has gone beyond the potential for relapse. This is the step all people who have com-menced action want to get to. Most people who have become a reg-ular exerciser want to remain one, indefinitely. Most people who have lost weight want to keep it off, permanently. Most people who have quit smoking want to be an exsmoker forever. Thus they have either permanently stopped engaging in a negative behavior such as cigarette smoking or eating a high-fat diet (that is *terminated* it), or, as in the case of regular exercise, *permanently* incorporated into their life a new, positive behavior, at least for the forseeable future.

Lapse may still occur, and in regular exercise, for example, as noted previously is actually a good idea periodically. Periodic lapse can also demonstrate that to stay in control over the long run, achieving perfection is absolutely not necessary. But *relapse* is not on the agenda.

It happens that for many, once the Permanent Maintenance stage is reached, the behavior itself, such as regular exercise, is found to be self-reinforcing. An outcome of behavior change, like being thinner or cough-free, can reinforce the behavior change as well. In the case of regular exercise, most who do it find that if they stop for too long, they just do not feel well, and are almost impelled to take up their activity(s) again. There are in fact some regular exercisers who because of this phenomenon find it difficult to take the occasional pause-for-recharging break that is beneficial for most.

Achieving Permanent Maintenance is thus the ultimate objective for implementing any of the Big Ten Set of Personal Health Promoting Behaviors and activities. Doing so marks the passing of a significant milestone on the wellness road. Staying with it, ensuring that the change is indeed permanent, is part of one's lifelong wellness journey. Essential to progress through the Stages of Change is the ability to mobilize motivation, the subject of Concept IX.

CONCEPT IX: MOTIVATION IS A PROCESS, NOT A THING

DEFINITION

Most people have a general idea of what they mean when they say "I've got to get motivated," or "my motivation is high for this one." But few of us can immediately put into words exactly what we mean when we use the term. Indeed, even among professionals, many who use it frequently don't bother to define it. Possibly this is so because it is assumed that everyone just *knows* how it is defined, even if that is often not the case. But because motivation is so important if success is to be achieved in behavior change, being familiar with a written definition is helpful. One approach is:

> Motivation is a mental process that links an emotion, feeling, desire, idea, or intellectual understanding, or a recognized psychological, physiological, or health need, to the taking of one or more actions.

In simpler terms, motivation is a process that connects a thought or a feeling to an action.

When we talk about either being motivated or lacking motivation to engage in a behavior change such as learning how to manage stress better or stop smoking, we are referring to the process of mind that will impel us to undertake that action (or, in the case of negative motivation, hinder us from doing so). Thus motivation is *always* related to action. (Note that the words motivation and move share the same Latin root.)

It is important to understand that motivation is not something tangible. It is not a thing that can or must be acquired somewhere or from someone else. It is, to repeat, an internal, mental, process. And in other than self-destructive persons, the process, even if inactive, is always present. For the striving to be healthy is essential both to self-preservation and species preservation. Thus getting motivated is not a matter of developing or importing a mind state. It is, rather, a matter of activating a process of the mind that is present but presently inoperative, of locating it, of mobilizing it, of removing barriers to its activation.

EXTERNAL VS. INTERNAL DIRECTION OF MOTIVATION

The scientific literature is clear that in most cases, if it is to be effective, motivation must be inner directed (Curry & Wagner, 1991; Curry, Wagner, & Grothaus, 1990). Thus, if the motivational process is to be effectively activated, there should be thoughts along the lines of: "I want to do this for me, to look better, feel better, get healthier, feel better about myself, for me, not for anyone else."

Externally originated motivation, "I'm doing this for my (spouse, significant other, boy/girl friend, children/parents, employer/coworkers)" almost invariably leads to one or more of: guilt feelings, anxiety, anger, frustration, and then, often, quitting (in Prochaska & DiClemente terms, Relapse). The one exception to the inner-directed rule is when the person can honestly say. "I'm doing this for someone else because it will make me feel good and feel good about myself to make them happy." But even in this case the primary motivation-mobilizer is still internal.

If one wants to look better, feel better, feel better about oneself, and get healthier, for oneself, for no one else, then one has inner motivation. If one views approval by others for making the behavior

change and achieving its desired outcome(s) simply as an extra benefit of doing so, then too does one have inner motivation. With inner
motivation it will be possible to take control of one's physical activity pattern and level, mode of eating, use of drugs such as nicotine
and alcohol, approach to managing stress, and so on and so forth
and to achieve health promoting/disease preventing changes in
one's body, one's self, and the way one lives one's life.

GUILT-FEELINGS AS A MOTIVATOR

When contemplating a positive lifestyle/behavior change, some
people have such thoughts as: "I *have* to," "I *ought* to," and "I *should*"
(in contrast with "I *want* to" and "I *would like* to"). "Have to," "ought
to," and "should" are all representations of a potential feeling of
guilt, that is "a painful feeling of self-reproach resulting from a belief
that one has done something wrong or immoral" (Webster's New
World Dictionary, 1970).

Much experience has shown that this guilt-inducing "you-gotta"
approach, whether self-inflicted or other inflicted, if it elicits guilt
feelings, has been generally found to be counterproductive. Thus
they don't work very well as a motivator (Miller & Rollnick, 1991).
Guilt feelings often elicit (in psychological terms) "resistance" or
"denial." In lay language, those terms translate as "I don't wanna,"
and "Problem? What problem?"

Furthermore, feeling guilty about anything without fairly quick
resolution of those feelings often leads to frustration and then anger.
Most of us don't like feeling either angry or frustrated on an ongoing basis. If feeling guilty is the reason we started doing it in the
first place, then the presence of those thoughts is likely to lead us
to quit doing what we're doing, for doing so will be the easiest way
to get rid of the anger and frustration.

However, let us assume that your client's motivation is positively
activated and that your client is working through the Preparation
Stage to the Action Stage. What are the practical steps required to
ensure that the behavior change process works? That is the subject
of Concept X.

CONCEPT X: ASSESSMENT, GOAL SETTING, AND MOBILIZING MOTIVATION ARE THE CENTRAL TASKS IN PERSONAL BEHAVIOR CHANGE

ASSESSMENT

At the outset there are two primary tasks to be undertaken to start right on the road to making any health-promoting behavior change: assessment and goal setting. These tasks are interconnected with one another and with the on-going process of behavior change in a continuous, self-reinforcing, feed-back loop. Assessment is of two types: self and health-professional. We will cover the former in this chapter, the latter in the next.

Self-assessment, as we shall see, is closely connected to goal setting. The elements of self-assessment are of the mind, of the body, and of one's previous experience. Your patients/clients need to take a clear look at their mental states if they are even in the Contemplation stage, considering such questions as:

- What is it that I am unhappy with (if anything)?
- What is it that I might/do want to change? And why? (This leads directly on to goal setting, see below.)
- Would I *really* like to change even if it means giving up something I'm accustomed to?
- Do I think that I can mobilize the mental strength to significantly change a personal behavior, if that is what I want/need to do?
- And (your client/patient should say to himself or herself), am I being realistic about this?

Concerning their body, the questions should be along the lines of:

- What is it that I like? Don't like? Would like to change?
- What is my body self-image, truly? Does it at all correspond to reality as others tell me that reality is?

Finally, what has their previous experience with personal health behavior change been? Good? Bad? Some success? None? Will that help this time round? What can be learned from past experience that will help this time?

Some people will want to complete a formal "Wellness Self-Assessment" questionnaire. Many have been written. Good ones can be found, for example, in Don Ardell's (1986) *High Level Wellness* (pp. 63–91, 309–320) and Carolyn Chambers Clark's (1996) *Wellness Practitioner*, 2nd ed. (pp. 27–29). They consider questions (each with many subquestions) like (Ardell, 1986, pp. 63–91):

- What is your level of self-responsibility?
- Do you engage in high-risk behaviors?
- What is your level of environmental sensitivity?
- Do you make appropriate use of the medical system?
- What is your level of nutritional awareness?
- What is your level of physical fitness?
- How are you at stress management?

SELF-IMAGE

As noted above, an important part of self-assessment is reviewing one's self-image. How does one think of oneself? Good-looking? Attractive? Not attractive? Healthy? Unhealthy? What does one see when one looks in the mirror? What kinds of feelings do those images elicit? And when one sees, for instance, "fat," do others say that that is a true reflection of reality? If your client is planning to exercise to help in weight-loss or simply shape up a currently out-of-shape body, will he or she be able to use clothing fit and the fact that his or her waist is getting smaller (that's at least small*er*, if not *small*) as measures of success, rather than something like scale weight (which might or might not change much, even as one is redistributing body mass)?

How much weight would have to be lost to get below the upper limit of the normal weight range for age, height, and sex? Would that make the person truly happier, or would your client feel the urge to lose even more weight? Is the true goal to become really *thin* rather than somewhat thinn*er*? Are they in reality looking for the "perfect body" (Brownell, 1991)? And if so, why? Answering these questions will be very important in mobilizing motivation and defining goals.

ASSESSING READINESS TO BEGIN

Most people will use both objective and subjective criteria in coming to the decision to begin a program of behavior change. Continuing to take an overweight person as the example, one objective criterion might be that measure of overall body size called the body mass index (BMI). It is a number derived from a formula that factors in both weight and height to represent a person's degree of fatness. An overweight person could, for example, find their BMI number on the BMI table, and if it were above normal could then decide to attempt to lose weight or body fat.

However, in reality, few overweight people would come to the conclusion that they are too heavy using such objective criteria alone, and thus decide to do something about it, really *do* something about it *this* time. That is, not too many people wake up one day, go to the BMI table, determine that their BMI is 10 units too high and then say, "OK, the time has come to lose some weight. Tomorrow I'm going to start a comprehensive program of regular exercise and healthy eating."

Much more likely is a scenario in which after quite some time of being overweight the person finally *feels*, deep down inside, that the time has come to lose weight, and, perhaps after a number of previous failures, is prepared to seriously attempt to do so, over an extended period of time. For example, such a person might say to themselves: "I'm just tired of being overweight and out of shape. I know how and why I got this way, and I have decided to take control of my body and my life. I'm finally going to do something about my weight and shape that will work in the long run. I know it's going to be tough, but I'm going to do it."

On the other hand, objective criteria such as dissatisfaction with being out-of-breath after climbing one flight of stairs, or the internalization of the relative risk in smokers of developing lung cancer, can lead one to becoming a regular exerciser or quitting cigarette use.

STARTING WHEN READY

Finally in self-assessment is the determination of when one is truly ready to start. A key to success is not starting until that point is reached. It involves a true understanding of the differences between Precontemplation, Contemplation, and Preparation before moving on to Action. This is one area where the health professional can be very helpful: making sure that that element of self-assessment is done and done accurately. Also critical is the decision to start, no less than the motivational process itself, to be effective must be inner generated. The person must both be and feel ready to go, within themselves, not because someone else (you, friend, or family) says they should.

In this regard, be sure to remember that the Concept of the Natural History of Health applies to everyone.

GOAL (AND OBJECTIVE) SETTING

Once the Contemplation Stage is reached, the single most important element of any personal behavior change undertaking is goal setting. For it is the process of goal setting that enables the Contemplators to focus, indeed forces them to focus, on the task at hand, to mobilize their motivation (see below) around self-established hoped-for outcomes that are realistic and meaningful for themselves. Through the medium of asking the questions "why," "why now," "what," and "what for?" these persons will lay the foundation for planning and organizing a specific behavior/ change program that is relevant to themselves and has meaning for themselves.

A goal is a general statement of a desired outcome: "I would like to learn how to handle my stress better. I would like to get my drinking under control." An objective is a specific measurable outcome that it is thought can be achieved within a specified period of time: "At the end of a month, I will be on a regular schedule of walking, 20 minutes per day, three times per week." (In this book, when the term "goal" is used, the term "objective" is subsumed under it.)

Goal setting and taking some time to do it forces the person to focus on the *reasons why* they want to change, not just the change process itself (as so many purely behavioral approaches do). *Goal setting is indeed the "magic wand" that clearly establishes the link between thought and action that is by definition the motivational process* (see the next section).

In helping patients and clients to set goals, it is essential for health professionals to help their patients and clients to address such questions as:

- What is it that you want to do?
- Why do you want to do it?
- What result are you looking for, for your efforts?
- For whom do you want to make the change(s), yourself or someone else?
- Do you want to feel better? Look better? Feel better about yourself? Reduce your future risk of disease? Become healthier?
- Are you being realistic about what you would like to accomplish?

It is important to stress, as discussed above under the Concept of motivation, if the goals set are internally, not externally, generated, the chances of quitting are significantly reduced, and the chances are significantly increased that the outcome of the person's efforts will be the happy, healthy, gradual, comfortable, incorporation of whatever the new element is into their life and lifestyle.

Goal setting will make it easier for the person to stick with the program when those "quitting thoughts" arise (and they invariably do). Because then it will not be simply "I've got to stick with this because I've got to stick this," but rather "I've got to stick with this for the reasons I started doing what I'm doing in the first place, and [hopefully] I very much still want to get where I originally decided I want to get to."

Goal setting provides the person with something to measure the outcome(s) of their efforts against. Finally, many of those who set out to make significant alterations in how they live their lives, and then fail to do so, neglected to clearly establish and delineate their goals (and to make sure that the goals set were reasonable ones for themselves, which thought leads to the next point).

REALISM

Realism in goal setting is essential. The initial goals set must be reasonable ones at the time they are set. It is important to recognize that what is "realistic" will likely change over time, if the behavior change/wellness process is truly engaged. It is important to remember that goals can always be changed to fit whatever the reality is at a given time. Thus, it is necessary to be very clear in one's head, not only what one wants to accomplish and why they want to accomplish it, but also that the goal set can be realistically reached. Nothing kills the change process better than the setting of unrealistic, unachievable goals.

Let us take regular exercise as an example. Speed, strength, muscular bulk, flexibility, gracefulness, are in part achieved through training and practice. However, the potential for achievement along these parameters is obviously in significant part determined by a person's genetic makeup. For each individual, exactly what proportion of each achievement is determined by their DNA structure and what proportion by their conscious effort is of course not as yet known. But few of us have the genetic makeup to enable us to be like either a world-class athlete or a world-class model, no matter how much work we do. Thus *not* setting goals of that sort, even in relative terms, will be liberating and empowering. Realism in goal setting will go a long way toward enhancing the chances of success in behavior change efforts.

Assessing Goal-Achievement

Goal achievement can be assessed subjectively and objectively. Among the questions that can be addressed to the change maker are:

- Have you achieved your goals and how well?
- Are your goals appropriate for you? If there is something wrong, is it with you or your goals?
- How's it going? Do you like what you are doing? If so, why, and if not, why not?
- Is it time to set new, more ambitious goals?
- Are perhaps the present ones too ambitious and in need of scaling back?
- Any injuries (in regular exercise), anger, frustration, guilt-feelings?
- In a regular exercise program again, is it possibly time to change sports or add a new one to a multisport program? Is it

time, perhaps, to take some time off, or cut back a bit in frequency or intensity?
- If weight-loss is the goal, has your weight changed? If it has gone up, is the increase due to adding body fat or adding muscle? If it has gone down, did the loss consist of body fat or muscle mass (the latter being unhealthy)?
- Are you feeling good and feeling good about yourself? (After all, that is, increasing self-esteem, may be the best measure of success of all.)

Periodic assessment of goal achievement and the goals themselves are an important part of that "continuous feed-back loop" of assessment/goal setting/reassessment/goal resetting that is so central to the behavior change process.

MOBILIZING MOTIVATION:
TAKING CONTROL; TAKING RESPONSIBILITY

How then do we go about getting through the stages of motivation and action described by Prochaska and DiClemente in practice, eventually reaching the stage of Permanent Maintenance? Occurring primarily in Stages 2 and 3 of the Prochaska and DiClemente model, there are four phases in "finding" or "developing" motivation:

1. Experiencing emotional or intellectual thought processes of the motivational type (as in the definition stated above).
2. Establishing a clear, open, unblocked mental pathway between those thoughts and the decision to begin taking the related action.
3. Setting one's goals, using the approach for so doing just described.
4. Taking the action as the result of activating one's motivation. Positive change does not occur without positive motivation.

"Taking control" is critical to locating/unblocking/mobilizing motivation. The persons say to themselves, "yes, I can do this, I can [for example,] run my eating pattern instead of having it run me." For many people, the mental act of "taking control" is itself a central element in both commencing a behavior change effort and in sticking with it. There are obviously many choices to make: *whether* to undertake a change process at all; *what* goals to set; how precisely to do it (e.g., what sort of exercise program to begin, what approach to weight-loss to use, whether to try to stop smoking "cold turkey" or through a program of gradual detoxification).

When a patient/client is in the contemplation or preparation stage, among other things they are engaged in the process of mobilizing their motivation. It is important to emphasize that motivation is almost always there in most people, whether or not it is currently activated. It is not a thing that one can import nor can someone else give it to someone. One has to unleash it within oneself. Only when the linkage between the thought or feeling on the one hand and the action on the other is made is motivation mobilized. And it is then, obviously, that one moves from contemplation to preparation and on to the action stage.

Among the common blocks to the motivation process that accompany so many attempts at behavior change are: "I really don't want to do this," "I know I'll just never be able to get started," "I just know I don't have the time." There is no magic answer for getting through these blocks, but *self*-assessment and goal setting, by the patients/clients themselves, certainly can help.

Taking control of one's body is an important aspect of this process, as noted. Taking control is empowering, as is the realization that one is taking control when perhaps one has not done that too often in the past. "Yes, I am doing this; yes, I can do this," whatever the "this" is, can bring joy and open up new vistas for many people. It certainly helps to keep them going. It can also help them deal with the fear of failure (Cooper, 1985).

Making choices, of course, means taking responsibility oneself, for oneself. Taking control and taking responsibility both are mental processes known to psychologists to be very powerful mobilizers of the motivational process.

AMBIVALENCE

Ambivalence can be a major factor inhibiting the mobilization of motivation. Ambivalence is a state of mind characterized by coexisting but conflicting feelings about a contemplated action, another person, or a situation in which one finds oneself (Miller and Rollnick, 1991). This state of mind often leads to a formulation such as: "I *want* to/I *don't* want to; I *know* I can do this/I really *don't think* I can do this;" "one day I want to and the next day I don't" (p. 38)

Feeling ambivalent from time to time is a perfectly healthy state of mind. Virtually everyone who even thinks about making a major (and sometimes even a minor) change in their lives experiences it. But to get on with the change process, ambivalence has to be dealt with. The inner conflict has to be resolved. Allowing it to paralyze decision-making is a problem. It is what one *does* in response to the feelings that determines their impact, of course.

Handled in the right way, the process of resolving ambivalent feelings itself can actually help in getting started down the road to success in changing a health-related behavior. The first key to effectively deal with ambivalence is to simply accept that it will always be present to some extent, and that's okay. Sometimes the ambivalent feelings will be weaker, sometimes stronger.

To get started your patient will have to be able to get at least partly on the track that already exists in his or her mind that leads to thoughts like "yes, I *would like to* change, yes I *can* change." Ambivalence does not have to be completely resolved to get started, however. Even as, for example, a regular exerciser may occasionally encounter negative feelings ranging from just not wanting to get out of bed in time to work out on a particular morning, to thinking "why am I doing this, anyway?" But then they continue, anyway.

Those sorts of thoughts are okay—as long as one doesn't get so far away from the program that what has already been accomplished is undone, and the stage of Relapse is entered. If ambivalence *destroys* commitment, that's a problem. However, if it simply *questions* commitment, if it does nothing more than lead to a temporary detour now and again, it can even be a good thing, leading to a strengthening of resolve to proceed forward. Again, as in motivation-mobilization, self-assessment and goal setting are powerful tools for dealing with ambivalence.

DEALING WITH THE NEED FOR IMMEDIATE GRATIFICATION

In contemporary American society, immediate gratification or the promise of it are common elements of our social consciousness.

Urgings to indulge in immediate gratification come at us in many forms and from many directions. For example, we have been told that if you have a sudden hunger for that certain burger, boy, you had better go right out and satisfy that hunger, right now. And we are told to do that regardless of what else is going on in our lives at the time.

Consider the problem in the weight loss context. We live in a weight loss environment that focuses on scale weight and its decline, *now*: "10 Lbs. in 7 Days" is the common supermarket tabloid headline. But it is well known in weight-loss science that that approach happens to be oh-so counter-productive in the long run. It almost invariably leads right into the "yo-yo dieting" trap. In the weight-loss context, how then does one deal with the problem of immediate gratification when for a variety of reasons significant and permanent weight loss is so difficult for so many to achieve and almost never happens overnight?

It is certainly possible to rationally understand where the drive for immediate gratification comes from and to know that it can only harm, not help. But in addition to, or in place of, that approach there is a kind of immediate gratification that can be obtained from the "taking control" process itself. It is a *mental* immediate gratification, not a physically measured one like scale weight. It is the immediate gratification that comes from self-empowerment, taking responsibility, doing something new and different.

If, for example, your client is able to start exercising regularly, even with short workouts three-to-four times per week, in less than a month or so, without any significant physical changes yet apparent, she may well start to think:

"Yes! I can *really* do this. I really can free up some time for myself, go outside, and go walking, on a weekly schedule. I can take control and make a positive change in my life, right now, and that feels good."

These kinds of thoughts may even occur during the preprogram planning phase (Contemplation/Preparation in the Prochaska & DiClemente terminology). That's immediate gratification of the positive kind.

ON WILLPOWER

And finally, on willpower. Given that willpower in terms of personal behavior means the *conscious mental ability* to follow through on plans to change it or to maintain a change once it is made, then willpower is absolutely essential to success. Don't let anyone or any book (like those "no willpower diet" ones) tell you or your patients/clients anything different. For in the context of one's personal health, "using willpower" simply *means* the mobilization of one's mental capacity to make a change in the carrying out of a physical act, like exercising/not exercising, eating/not eating a healthy diet, smoking/not smoking cigarettes. Nothing more; nothing less. And that is precisely what the personal behavior change-maker needs to do to make the desired change(s).

It's that simple, and that complicated; it's that easy, and that difficult. But that, at the center, is what both the process Concepts approach to personal behavior change and the Stages of Change themselves are all about: using one's willpower to get on and stay on the wellness pathway.

REFERENCES

Ardell, D. B. (1986). *High level wellness: An alternative to doctors, drugs and disease*. Berkeley, CA: Ten Speed Press.

Brownell, K. D. (1991). Dieting and the Search for the Perfect Body. *Behavior Therapy, 22*, 1–12.

Clark, C. C. (1996). *Wellness practitioner: Concepts, research and strategies*. New York: Springer Publishing.

Cooper, K. (1985). *Running without fear*. New York: M. Evans and Co.

Curry, S. J., & Wagner, E. H. (1991). Evaluation of intrinsic and extrinsic motivation interventions with a self-help smoking cessation program. *Journal of Consulting and Clinical Psychology, 59*, 318.

Curry, S. J., Wagner, E. H., & Grothaus, L. C. (1990). Intrinsic and extrinsic motivation for smoking cessation. *Journal of Consulting and Clinical Psychology, 58*, 310–316.

Heatherton, T. F., & Tickle, J. (1999). Exploding the Myth: Dieting Makes You Thin. *Healthy Weight Journal, 13*, 7.

Miller, W. R., & Rollnick, S. (1991). *Motivational interviewing: Preparing people to change addictive behavior* (pp. 5–7). New York: The Guilford Press.

Polivy, J. (1999). The Mythology of Dieting. *Healthy Weight Journal, 13,* 1.

Prochaska, J. O. (1993). Working in Harmony with How People Change Naturally. *The Weight Control Digest, 3,* 249.

Prochaska, J. O., & DiClemente, C. C. (1982). Transtheoretical therapy: Toward a more integrative model of change. *Psychotherapy: Theory, Research, and Practice, 19,* 276–288.

Prochaska, J. O., DiClemente, C. C., & Norcross, J. C. (1992). In Search of How People Change: Applications to Addictive Behavior. *American Psychologist, 47,* 1102–1114.

Prochaska, J. O., Norcross, J. C., & DiClemente, C. C. (1992). Attendance and Outcome in a Worksite Weight Control Program: Processes and Stages of Change as Process and Predictor Variables. *Addictive Behaviors, 17,* 35–45.

Prochaska, J. O., & Velicer, W. F. (1997). The Transtheoretical Model of Behavior Change. *American Journal of Health Promotion, 12,* 38–48.

Velicer, W. F., & Prochaska, J. O. (1997). Introduction: The Transtheoretical Model. *American Journal of Health Promotion, 12,* 6.

United States Preventive Services Task Force. (1989). *Guide to Clinical Preventive Services,* Baltimore, MD: Williams and Wilkins.

Webster's new world dictionary, Second College Edition. (1970). New York: The World Publishing Co.

USING THE TEN CENTRAL CONCEPTS IN CLINICAL PRACTICE

III

USING THE TEN CENTRAL CONCEPTS IN CLINICAL PRACTICE: GENERAL CONSIDERATIONS

I. THE TEN CENTRAL CONCEPTS REVIEWED

In this chapter, I continue the general discussion of how to use the Ten Central Concepts of Health Promotion/Disease Prevention (HP/DP) in clinical practice with patients and clients. In the next chapter, I shall look at their use in a specific setting: helping a patient or client to become a regular exerciser.

To review, the Ten Central Concepts are:

I. Health is a state of being; wellness is a process of being.
II. Health status is determined by a broad range of factors.
III. Health has a natural history.
IV. Central to the wellness process is a wide array of HP/DP interventions.
V. Success in certain behavior change endeavors is relative.
VI. Risks to health can be reduced; in few instances is there certainty of outcome.
VII. Achieving balance is the essence of healthy living and wellness.

VIII. There is a common pathway to success for most personal
behavior change efforts.
IX. Motivation is a process, not a thing.
X. Assessment, goal setting, and mobilizing motivation are the
central tasks in personal behavior change.

The process Concepts discussed in the previous chapter describe
the routes followed to get to a healthy/well state of being, using
the seven substantive Concepts discussed in chapter 4 to inform the
process. Since chapter 5 is already heavily focussed on the application of the three process Concepts in clinical practice, in this chapter, I shall explore further the application in practice of the
substantive Concepts, I–VII.

I. HEALTH IS A STATE OF BEING;
WELLNESS IS A PROCESS OF BEING

Although patients, the media, and even some health professionals
use the terms interchangeably, as we have seen health and wellness
are not the same thing. That health is a state of being and wellness
a process of being is not some arcane academic conceit, however,
because to live a long, happy, productive life requires both: Being
measurably healthy at given points in time *and* being on the wellness pathway over time. When it is explained to them, many
patients and clients will find the distinction between the two useful in helping them to plan their own futures.

On a number of occasions the view has been expressed in this
book that wellness goes well beyond health to deal with such areas
of being as joy, creativity, productivity, intellectual fulfillment, societal responsibility, and its expression. Without using the precise
term, Dr. Lester Breslow (1999) refers to it as: "[T]he energy and
reserves of health that permit a buoyant life, full of zest and the
eager ability to meet life's challenges. . . . (p. 1032)"

Our old friend Dr. Don Ardell (1999), who has offered numerous
characterizations of wellness, a number of them presented in chapter 2, further has this to say:

Wellness is a term for thinking of health from a performance point
of view. It is a perspective, a mindset or a way of looking at per-

formance realities. Wellness entails a disciplined, conscious pursuit of a dynamic state of physical and psychological well being beyond the mediocrity of normal non-sickness or the standard level of dysfunctional mindsets. . . .

Wellness is a lifestyle approach to personal excellence, to a life that celebrates personal freedom, good health, the search for meaning and purpose, humor, adventure and all that is within our power or reach that seems positive, moral, worthy and of consequence. (p. 1)

If you agree with the view that wellness goes well beyond health you should share that view with your patients/clients.

II. HEALTH STATUS IS DETERMINED BY A BROAD RANGE OF FACTORS

That health status at any one time is determined by a group of factors and influences, not just one, is important in the clinical practice of health promotion/disease prevention for several reasons. First, if clients or patients think that they are "not doing anything about their health right now," they may be pleasantly surprised to find that indeed they are, without recognizing it. So, an overweight, inactive, nonsmoker is still a nonsmoker. An uptight executive who never fastens his automobile seatbelt but who is of normal weight and drinks no more than an occasional glass of wine at dinner, is still a nonobese, nonabuser of alcohol.

Many people who want to do something about their health think that they are presently doing nothing and thus facing a daunting task. However, given Concept II, the message you can give such people is usually of the "you are already on the wellness pathway; you simply have to consider if you want to do more" type, not the "boy, it will be tough; you're starting from ground-zero" one. Second, some people come to the wellness pathway with built-in health status advantages, like a genetically determined low blood pressure or no family history of cancer. Having such a "leg up" can be cheering and encouraging.

Third, it is important for patients to recognize that even if they are on the wellness pathway, being and staying healthy is not entirely their personal responsibility. Among that "broad range of factors" are many environmental as well as genetic ones that are beyond their control. It will be very helpful for most people to learn to control what they can control (including their responses to external factors) and give up trying to control what they cannot (that is, many of those external factors). That in itself is a very important element of healthy living.

The common theme of these observations is that we don't want people to get mentally weighed down by thinking that the task of being personally well and staying healthy is so enormous that it is not even worth trying. Yes, if you are getting the impression that among our most important functions as health professionals are: encouragement of change, endorsement of the idea that most of us have within us resources of which we are not presently aware, enhancement of most people's inherent will to be healthy, and being cheerleaders for health and wellness and the ability of most people to lead healthier lives once they can mobilize their motivation to do so—you're right!

III. HEALTH HAS A NATURAL HISTORY

This Concept is closely connected with both Concept I and Concept II. Health status changes over time. When it moves or is kept moving in a positive direction it can be said that the person is engaged in the wellness process. It is the very rare person indeed who can be entirely healthy, can "do everything right," can have all of their controllable risk factors under the best control at all times. But, as noted, most people do certain things "right" and have at least some of the controllable personal risk factors highlighted by the "Big Ten" list under control at any given time.

Equally important in helping patients and clients to get well and stay well is the knowledge that where control of a personal health behavior is not being undertaken by a given person at a given time, that doesn't mean that they might be able to do so 6 months from now, 1 year from now, 5 years from now. And "that's okay" is the message to transmit to patients. Health care professionals need to let them know, over and over again, that with a few exceptions (see below under Concept VII) perfection isn't the objective here, that different people change at different rates of speed, and that even though they may not be ready or able to—lose weight, start exercising, give up smoking cigarettes—*now*, if they are like everybody else, they may very well be able to do it down the road, when *they* are ready.

For example:

- They may be able to do it because over time they will rationally think their way to the moment of change: "OK, if I keep drinking like I'm drinking now, and have been for the last 10 years, I'm surely going to kill myself early, and I may end up killing someone else too. So I had better stop, right now."
- They may do it because of an external event that hits home: a dear aunt who was a life-long smoker dies a very uncomfortable, premature death from chronic obstructive pulmonary disease (and just after that event your client quits using cigarettes).
- Like the man who started exercising regularly after being out-of-breath at the top of that ramp in Detroit's Cobo Hall (see chapter 4, p. 56), on a given day, for temporal reasons not at all understood, your patient may experience a specific health-related "learning moment" that changes their life.

IV. CENTRAL TO THE WELLNESS PROCESS IS A BROAD ARRAY OF HP/DP INTERVENTIONS

Just as there is a spectrum of factors influencing health, so is there an array of personal interventions that one can undertake on the wellness pathway to improve it. Once again, it is important for the clinician to maintain a positive message for the Contemplator of HP/DP behavior change:

- "One step at a time."
- "If that one (weight loss) is too difficult, why not try that one (becoming a regular exerciser without attempting to lose weight)."
- "If you are an overweight, sedentary smoker, and it all seems overwhelming, why not start out with something that might be easier, such as attending to personal safety issues like fastening your seatbelt every time you get in the car, or attending to your immunization status."

In facilitating positive behavior change, it can be extremely helpful to patients and clients to know that they have choices, that the choices are theirs to make, that some choices are easier to implement than others, and that it's okay to start out with the easier ones.

Suppose you have a client who has done little yet to improve his health over the course of his lifetime and cannot be considered to be on the wellness pathway. He tells you that he would somehow like to get on it, but is feeling rather overwhelmed with the seeming enormity of the task. Doing something relatively simple like the aforementioned fastening of his seatbelt every time he gets into his car may be what it takes to show him that, yes, he can take control of his behavior in at least one venue, yes, he can do something to get a major risk factor under control, and, yes, if he can take control of that behavior, maybe, just maybe, he can take on something rather more difficult, like cutting down on the amount of fat in his diet.

V. SUCCESS IN CERTAIN BEHAVIOR CHANGE ENDEAVORS IS RELATIVE

Again in terms of facilitation of positive behavior change, of helping clients/patients to overcome mental barriers to change, of making changes appear to be doable for each client, in dealing with behaviors for which an absolute outcome—*not* using tobacco products, *not* abusing alcoholic beverages—it is important to stress the idea that the goals they set must be appropriate and realistic. The definition of success for patients and clients is of course entirely interlinked with the goal(s) they have set for themselves. Once goals are realistically delineated, then what constitutes success can be realistically delineated as well.

First, what constitutes success varies from person to person. Second, and this is part of the natural history of health, within each person what constitutes success can vary over time, too. Recall the saying "explore your limits; recognize your limitations." This has particular applicability to the concept that what is success is relative. Exploring one's limits, gradually and realistically, especially in the arena of regular exercise, can lead one to achievements not previously contemplated. Examples of the relativity of success were presented in the consideration of this concept in chapter 4.

VI. RISKS TO HEALTH CAN BE REDUCED; IN FEW INSTANCES IS THERE CERTAINTY OF OUTCOME

This is something of a negative that health professionals need to deal with in talking with patients about health promotion and disease prevention. In health terms, the only guarantee that can be given to a person who loses weight, who becomes a regular exerciser, who stops smoking cigarettes, is that they will have reduced their chances of coming down with one or more of the diseases or negative health conditions associated with obesity, sedentary lifestyle, and tobacco use, respectively. However, there is and can be no guarantee that the person will *not* develop diabetes, die of a heart attack, or contract lung cancer.

On the other hand, we *can, virtually,* make *certain* guarantees. Let's say that your patient or client takes control, makes positive HP/DP changes in lifestyle, in a way and at a pace that make sense for the client and where the client is coming from, and gets on the wellness pathway and determines to stay on it. Almost every time, in the near future that person will feel better and will feel better about themselves, and may very well look better, too, if the change involved exercise, eating, or substance use/abuse, regardless of what might or might not happen in terms of specific diseases down the road of life. This all has to be clearly explained to clients and patients.

VII. ACHIEVING BALANCE IS THE ESSENCE OF HEALTHY LIVING AND WELLNESS

It is important to share with clients and patients the several different meanings of "balance" central to this Concept, again in aid of helping them to make positive behavior change(s). "Balance" first refers to balance within their lives at the present time, balance between work, play, and family. As Arnold and Breen (1998), citing Halbert Dunn, say: "[W]ell-being implies being well not only in the body and mind but also within the family and community and having a compatible work interest" (p. 5).

"Balance" also refers to balance in one's own efforts to get on and stay on the wellness road, engaging in HP/DP activities, among other things. As the ad says, "Just do it." But at the same time, be sure not to *over*do it. In health promotion, as noted, perfection is to be sought in certain areas: *not* using tobacco products; not *a*busing alcohol or any of the other recreational mood-altering drugs; *not* using prescription psychoactive drugs on a nonprescription basis; *always* practicing safe sex; and *maintaining* a healthy immune status. However, as for the other major arenas of HP/DP, weight, diet, physical activity, maintenance of personal safety, and stress management, it is always possible to overdo it. That must be avoided.

Balance is also to be sought in the speed at which behavior change is undertaken. Recall the saying "gradual change leads to permanent changes." The way to achieve successful weight loss is of course the prime example of the truth of this maxim. But it is equally critical to long-term success in regular exercise and dietary change without weight loss as the goal not to attempt to do too much too soon.

Finally, balance refers to the balance between personal health promoting measures and those related to the environment, discussed previously in chapter 2. In this regard, Dr. Lester Breslow (1999) quoted the Ottawa Charter for Health Promotion, sponsored by the World Health Organization: "[T]he fundamental conditions and resources for health are peace, shelter, education, food, income, a stable eco-system, sustainable resources, social justice and equity" (p. 1030). It should be noted that for the vast majority of the world's population these conditions and resources of course have been unobtainable under any socioeconomic system developed to date.

On the subject of balance Dr. Breslow goes on to refer to a "publication of the International Epidemiological Association and the World Health Organization" as describing two aspects of health: health balance and health potential. He summarizes their view as:

> Health balance is essentially the Hippocratic notion [see also chapter 2 of this book] of dynamic equilibrium between the human organism and its environment, a basically stable relationship of a person with the world outside. On the other hand, health potential consists of reserves—an individual's capacity to cope with environmental influences that jeopardize health balance. This concept goes beyond the idea of immunity to harmful microbiological agents; it includes the capacity for withstanding the adverse effects of the factors causing atherosclerosis, the loss of a loved one, or myriad other injurious circumstances of living. (p. 1031)

Finally, Dr. Breslow says:

Accepting that health means both (1) the current state of a human organism's equilibrium with the environment, often called *health status*, and (2) the potential to maintain that balance, health promotion aims to *maintain and expand* human functioning . . . [it] means facilitating at least the maintenance of a person's current position on the [health] continuum and, ideally, advancing towards its positive end [emphasis added]" (p. 1032)

And that process, we may add, is what in this book we refer to as *wellness*.

And now let us turn to a consideration of some specific techniques to use in talking to and working with patients and clients on health promotion and disease prevention. This next section draws heavily on the work of Drs. Jane Westberg and Hilliard Jason (1996).

II. SOME TECHNIQUES FOR USING THE TEN CONCEPTS IN THE CLINICAL SETTING

A. TASKS AND ELEMENTS

The primary functions of the health professional during the encounter with an individual client/patient are:

A. Assessing
B. Evaluating
C. Educating
D. Recommending
E. Prescribing (limited applications in HP/DP)
F. Facilitating

Important elements in promoting health and getting on/staying on the wellness pathway beyond these primary functions are:

- Enhancing vitality
- Promoting self-discipline
- Authorizing self-empowerment

- Encouraging self-responsibility
- Eliciting creativity
- Enabling relaxation
- Removing barriers to change
- Improving communication skills
- Envisioning desired outcomes
- Taking full responsibility* for yourself

B. COLLABORATION VS. DIRECTION

"Educating," "recommending," "facilitating," "enhancing," "encouraging," "enabling," and so forth are verbs not so frequently seen as describing what health professionals do. But they are at the center of the role that works best in working with clients/patients on health promotion, disease prevention, and getting on/staying on the wellness pathway: the collaborative role.

The essence of that role is helping patients and clients to find for themselves the answers they need to find rather than trying to tell them what to do. That role contemplates suggesting (recommending) rather than directing (prescribing). That role is facilitating rather than formulating. That role is sharing the power with patients rather than keeping it all for oneself and being willing to give it *all* away to patients/clients who demonstrate that they can take it and use it effectively.

While developing a collaborative rather than the traditional directive relationship with patients and clients would have benefit throughout the whole range of health care from health promotion/disease prevention through treatment to rehabilitation, it has special application to the subject at hand. First, in personal HP/DP for the most part patients and clients in the end have to do whatever they need to do for themselves. What better way to accomplish this end than by having them actively involved in the process with you from the beginning?

---

* As with Dr. Ardell on wellness (see chapter 2), that responsibility is limited to those factors affecting one's health that one can be reasonably expected to take responsibility for.

Second, the evidence is clear that the authoritative approach doesn't work nearly as well as the collaborative one (Westberg and Jason, 1996, p. 146). "Telling" just doesn't do the trick. Recall that an important element in mobilizing the motivational process is taking control. Another way of putting that is to say that we are "giving ownership" of the process to the patient or client.

Collaboration means involving patients in decision-making. It means facilitating but not trying to direct the Stages of Change process. It means presenting questions, not answers. To repeat, it means offering choices, not trying to make them for patients and clients. We empower clients and patients when we lay out for them to consider (and hopefully incorporate into their own thinking) what Westberg and Jason (1996) describe as the "steps to change" (p. 147). These, of course, occur through and with the Prochaska & DiClemente Stages of Change:

1. Acknowledging that something is not right in our lives.
2. Deciding that we want to make a change in our lives.
3. Doing an assessment and setting goals.
4. Exploring options for achieving them.
5. Deciding on a plan and implementing it.

Patience is an important characteristic of the successful clinician in this arena. Think "Natural History of Health" and "gradual change leads to permanent changes." Remember, your own behavior in the realm of patient/client behavior change is very important. There are many nonverbal messages, positive and negative, that are transmitted in the course of an encounter. (Role-modeling, one aspect of clinician behavior, is considered in some detail in chapter 7.)

One caveat. While promoting the collaborative approach, make sure that the particular patient/client wants it and, in your estimation, would benefit from it. Some folks are, indeed, more comfortable in a directive relationship. The latter is the one that is obviously more comfortable for any health professional who has been trained in it. In dealing with someone who you think wants and can benefit from direction rather than collaboration, just make sure that you are not projecting your traditional way of functioning onto them.

C. TALKING POSITIVELY

It is important to use nonthreatening language. Be sure to avoid putting your patients/clients on the defensive. You want to help them get to new stages in their lives. Forcing them, even unintentionally, to defend where they are now is distinctly not helpful. Equally unhelpful is running guilt trips on them. As discussed at some length in chapter 5, guilt feelings are a poor motivator. In fact, in the HP/DP context, having them or eliciting them is often counterproductive.

Recognize your patient's/client's past history and [hopefully] positive experiences with at least some elements of HP/DP and use them as they apply to the present situation. Many patients and clients, and family-members and friends of theirs as well, have previous experiences that can be very helpful in getting the person on the wellness pathway and staying there. Personal experiences of your own can be helpful as well (again, see the section on Role Modeling in chapter 7).

One way to use all past lessons, both positive and negative ones, is to have the person group them into "facilitating" and "obstructing." Then they will be able to clearly see what they did right and what they did wrong, and which external factors helped and hindered them. In helping patients/clients to get started, facilitating are such questions as:

- "Are you ready to . . . ?"
- "If not, why do you think you aren't . . . ?
- "Have you given any further thought to . . . ?"

Encourage patients to contribute their own ideas on moving through the Stages of Change and climbing the Steps of Change listed at the beginning of this section: goal setting, program design, and mobilizing their motivation. Self-assessment, discussed in the previous chapter, is very helpful in this process.

Finally, family members presently can be both helpful and hindering. For a full treatment of the potential positive role of family members, see, for example, *Help Your Man Get Healthy* (Kassberg & and Jonas, 1999).

III. HEALTH PROFESSIONAL ASSESSMENT

A. Dealing with Disease/Risk Factors

While patient/client self-assessment is central to success in HP/DP, health professional assessment is often important, too. The Big Ten Set of Personal Health Promoting Behaviors/Activities deal with factors in risk reduction for a host of major disease and negative health conditions. For example, as most of the readers of this book will know, several major diseases and medical conditions such as coronary artery disease, hypertension, osteoporosis, and noninsulin dependent diabetes, are associated with a sedentary lifestyle. Thus a program of regular exercise is useful in reducing the risk for acquiring them.

However, if your client/patient already has one or more certain diseases, possibly without being aware of that fact, and that person becomes a regular exerciser, in certain circumstances they will stand an increased risk of the occurrence of a harmful event. Thus, again for example, before starting a regular exercise program, either for its own sake or as part of a weight-loss program, if there is a history of any of the following diseases or conditions, you should recommend a thorough medical evaluation.

1. *A disease or condition associated with a clear risk of harm occurring during regular exercise*
   a. Previous myocardial infarction
   b. Chest pain, pressure in the chest, or severe shortness of breath upon exertion
   c. Any history of lung disease, especially chronic obstructive pulmonary disease
   d. Any bone, joint, or other disease or limitation affecting the muscles or skeletal system

2. *A disease or condition associated with a possibly elevated risk harm occurring during regular exercise*
   a. High serum cholesterol
   b. Cigarette smoking
   c. Hypertension

d. Abuse of drugs or alcohol
e. Prescribed medication used on a regular basis
f. Any other chronic illness, such as diabetes

B. HEALTH RISK APPRAISAL

In addition to engaging in what is essentially medical history taking for the identification of potentially harmful existing diseases
and conditions, health professionals can also undertake what is
generically referred to as "Health Risk Appraisal" (HRA) (Beery, et
al. 1986; Office of Disease Prevention and Health Promotion, 1986).
According to Beery and colleagues, health risk appraisal is:

> [A] health promotion technique in which a person's health-related
> behavior and personal characteristics are compared with mortal-
> ity statistics and epidemiological data. From this analysis are
> derived estimates of the risk of dying in the next 10 years, or at a
> particular age, as well as estimates of the amount of risk that could
> be eliminated by appropriate behavioral changes."

HRA uses a questionnaire that is customarily completed by the
patient or client and then scored by computer. It can be very helpful if the results then are discussed with and interpreted for the person by a health professional. HRA can be usefully employed with
the much more broadly focussed and self-administered/self-scored
"Wellness Appraisals" of the Ardell and Clark type referred to in
chapter 5 (p. 76). Numerous health risk appraisal instruments have
been developed over the years. The Office of Disease Prevention
and Health Promotion, the National Health Information Center, and
the Center for Disease Control and Prevention, divisions of the
Department of Health and Human Services in Washington, can provide information on the current roster of HRAs.

C. STAGES AND STEPS

Perhaps the most important part of health professional assessment
in health and wellness is helping your patients and clients determine just where they are on the Stages of Change continuum. Doing

so will help you and them to more sharply define their tasks, whether they be assessment, goal setting, mobilization of motivation, program planning, "getting on with it," dealing with lapse-relapse, and so on and so forth. The Prochaska & DiClemente Stages of Changes describe how one can and how one does climb the Westberg and Jason "steps to change." And that's what it's all about, isn't it?

As the saying goes: "If you are open to growth, you will always grow; if you are open to learning, you will always learn." Facilitating those processes is how we can help our clients and patients best.

REFERENCES

Ardell, D. (1999). *Ardell Wellness Report, 53,* 1.

Arnold, J., & Breen, L. J. (1998). Images of Health. In S. S. Gorin, & J. Arnold (Eds.), *Health promotion handbook.* St. Louis, MO: Mosby.

Beery, W., Schaerbach, U. J., Wagner, E. H., and associates. (1986). *Health risk appraisal: Methods and programs, with annotated bibliography.* Rockville, MD: National Center for Health Services Research and Health Care Technology Assessment. (DHHS Pub. No. [PHS] 86-3396).

Breslow, L. (1999). From Disease Prevention to Health Promotion. *Journal of the American Medical Association, 281,* 1030–1033.

Kassberg Regan, M., & Jonas, S. (1999). *Help your man get healthy.* New York: Whole Care/Avon.

Office of Disease Prevention and Health Promotion. (1986). *Integration of risk factor interventions: Two reports of the office of disease prevention and health promotion.* Washington, DC: US Dept. of Health and Human Welfare.

Westberg, J., & Jason, H. (1996). Influencing health behavior: The process. In S. H. Woolf, S. Jonas, & R. Lawrence (Eds.). *Health promotion and disease prevention in clinical practice.* Baltimore, MD: Williams and Wilkins.

Chapter 7

AN EXAMPLE: EXERCISE PROMOTION

INTRODUCTION

This chapter is about how to apply the Ten Central Concepts of health promotion/disease prevention (HP/DP) to a specific clinical situation. The example chosen is helping a patient or client to become, be, or become once again, a regular exerciser.* Those of the Ten Central Concepts that apply in this instance are woven throughout the chapter, thus highlighting, among other things, the existence of the single common pathway to most personal health promoting behavior change; and its utility in helping patients and clients to make disease preventive/health promotive change(s) in their lives.

One disclaimer. The principles for helping people to alter the way they live their lives in relation to health are the same whether we

---

* For a comprehensive approach to the subject of promoting regular exercise in clinical practice, you might want to refer to my book *Regular Exercise: A Handbook for Clinical Practice*, and its companion, abridged version, written for use by patients, *A Guidebook for the Regular Exerciser*. They were both published by Springer Publishing Co. in 1995.

are dealing with ill or otherwise healthy persons. But the application of the approach to regular exercise presented here is to the sedentary person who wants to exercise; the sedentary person who needs to exercise for risk factor modification; and the former or present exerciser who is looking for advice because of injury, burn-out, or a need for reinforcement. It is not intended as a primer for the use of regular exercise in either disease treatment or rehabilitation. That subject is best left in the hands of the specialist.

GETTING STARTED

FIRST STEPS

The first step in helping patients and clients to undertake most personal HP/DP behavior changes is to introduce them to the common factors in the process: assessment, goal setting, and mobilizing motivation (Concept X).

ASSESSMENT

For the details, please refer back to chapter 5. But there are a few points to emphasize in the context of working with patients and clients on regular exercise. Regular exercise by definition requires the commitment of time on a regular basis for as long as the person engages in the activity. That is a significant commitment, especially for busy people.

Thus it is especially important to introduce the Prochaska and DiClemente "Stages of Change Model" that is at the center of Concept VIII (see also chapter 5). You will find patients and clients all along the Stages continuum. But it is important for the persons themselves to understand the difference between precontemplation, contemplation, and preparation, and to be able to assess for themselves just where they are on the road to the action Stage.

Next in this context, remember that guilt is a poor motivator. If someone thinks that they are at the preparation stage or even the action stage, when they are really still in precontemplation or contemplation, and then gets all caught up in "why can't I do this, I must be a bad person" thoughts, that is obviously counterproductive. In such cases, you want to help the person focus on internally-supported self-assessment as the essential step to goal setting.

Concept III, "health has a natural history," can be helpful in discussing the Stages of Change, and so forth. For the patient/client leading a sedentary lifestyle, engaging in no job-related or leisure-time extraneous physical exertion, exercising regularly is obviously the only way to address that situation from the health perspective. But can one say, at any given time in life, "OK, I'm going to start a program now, I will stick with it indefinitely, and a lifetime pattern of regular exercise will be the result," and be assured of success? For most people, the answer to that question is "no."

Using Concept III you can then reassure the person that it's alright not to be ready right now, that the time is obviously not right for them, but that it may well be 6 months or even 2 years from now. And they will know when it is the right time, when they indeed have mobilized their motivation, with you there to help them.

For regular exercise, a special assessment issue concerns cardiac stress testing. For some years certain exercise authorities recommended that virtually all persons embarking on regular exercise programs first undergo cardiac stress testing (Cooper, 1985, 1994). In recent years, this has been modified. The current recommendation of the American College of Sports Medicine (ACSM) and the Cooper Institute (ACSM, 1999) is that when contemplating a program of vigorous exercise, apparently healthy males over 40 and females over 50 and any individuals with increased risk of cardiopulmonary or metabolic disease should undergo a maximal treadmill exercise test. So should, according to the ACSM, all persons with diseases on the ACSM list who are contemplating any kind of exercise program.

However, according to the *Guide to Clinical Preventive Services* of the U.S. Preventive Services Task Force (USPSTF) of the United States Public Health Service, there is no clear, statistically supported evidence that for an adult with no evidence of underlying heart disease, the performance of either a resting or treadmill exercise electrocardiogram is either necessary or useful in reducing the risk of an untoward outcome from exercising regularly (USPSTF, 1996 pp. 3–10). There is one exception to that rule, according to the USPSTF. Members of that group of males over 40 who have two or more risk factors for coronary artery disease other than sedentary lifestyle itself (such as elevated serum cholesterol, a history of cigarette smoking, hypertension, diabetes mellitus, or a family history of early-onset coronary artery disease), should have a cardiac stress test before beginning an exercise program.

GOAL SETTING

Recall that goal setting is the single most important element of any behavior change endeavor (Concept X). It encompasses knowing what one wants to do, why one wants to do it, for whom one is doing it, and what one expects to get out of it. The process has been covered at some length in chapter 5. We will review here a couple of the most important points that have a special application to exercise.

In setting exercise goals, realism is very important. An understanding of the relativity of success in this behavior change and of achieving balance (Concepts V and VII) is what one is looking for (see also below). At the outset, setting exercise goals that are truly beyond most people's abilities ("starting from scratch as a runner, within 3 months I will run a marathon"), will almost invariably lead to frustration, pain, injury, and quitting. If on the other hand, setting goals that are too low ("For as long as I exercise regularly, I will only walk, only at my regular walking pace, and for not more than 20 minutes at a time") will almost invariably lead to boredom and then failure to achieve any of the desired physical and mental outcomes of regular exercise.

At the same time, it's important to emphasize that goals can, and in many cases should, be changed over time. But that should be done gradually and realistically. There is potential magic in this: some people discover within themselves predilections and abilities they never previously had an inkling of.

As discussed earlier (also see chapter 5), the role of genes in determining what one can do must be recognized, again especially when it comes to exercise. There is that strong genetic component in, for example, the determination of body shape and size, potential strength, whether one can significantly increase muscle bulk by weight lifting, and speed in any sport. Goals should be suitably tailored to genetic realities.

Let's say that at the beginning a goal of doing a 10-kilometer ("10k," 6.2 mile) running road race is set. Unless your client is naturally fast, for the first one at least it is a good idea to define "doing" as "finishing the race" rather than "finishing in under 46 minutes" or "placing in my age-class." Once having achieved the goal of finishing a 10k and in the process getting some idea of what one's natural speed is—64 minutes rather than 46 may have proved to be it—appropriate speed goals for future races can then be set.

The same reasoning applies to distance goals that might be established. For the beginning regular runner interested in recreational racing, for example, it is highly advisable to think "5k" as a goal before thoughts of 10k, half-marathon, and marathon appear. Remember, as long as *limitations* are recognized, say in terms of speed, exploration of what one's true limits are, say in terms of distance, may lead into territory that has never before been contemplated, even in the wildest of dreams. The saying "gradual change leads to permanent changes" certainly has application here.

FEAR OF FAILURE

In some people this is an important element to take into account in goal setting. While that fear often has psychological roots that we have neither the time nor space to consider here, in some persons it can dealt with behaviorally. Setting doable goals and thinking about small steps—once again, "gradual change leads to permanent changes"—can be useful. If you can help your patients/clients to set short-term goals that they have a good chance of achieving, in series, that will increase their chances of staying with it.

Further, an important aspect of the goal setting process is the understanding that for many people regular exercise first and foremost means feeling good and feeling good about themselves *now*. For many people starting out, those feelings can arrive in a few weeks, regardless of how fast or how long they are going. As noted earlier, that psychological immediate gratification can be a powerful mobilizer of motivation and help many a person deal with fear of failure on the "objective" measures of exercise success.

FINDING THE TIME/MAKING THE TIME

As noted above, it is a fact of life that becoming a regular exerciser is time intrusive on the rest of one's life, *for* the rest of one's life. In this regard exercising regularly differs from most of the other primary personal lifestyle and behavior changes that promote health, for example, smoking cessation, substance abuse control, managing weight, changing eating habits, wearing one's automobile seatbelt. Unless the particular lifestyle change requires ongoing participation in, say, a 12-step or similar program, only regular exercise requires a significant amount of extra time, forever.

That time may be only 2 or 3 hours per week for exercising itself, plus another hour or 3 for changing clothes, showering, getting to the pool or gym. But those are 3 to 6 hours per week now being spent doing something else. This aspect of the enterprise should not be swept under the rug. It needs to be examined carefully.

How is time being spent now? Can your client or patient give up 4 hours of TV a week? Get up 45 minutes earlier 4 days per week (including the 2 weekend days) and cut down on dawdling time by 15 minutes on each of those days? Can a spouse, for example, do some of the food shopping and cooking and help with some household chores? If necessary, can some time be found during the work day to squeeze in time for training? Better yet, can advantage be taken of a health promotion program that many employers now sponsor, or can a suggestion be made to do so if one is not presently offered at the workplace?

A modestly demanding program of regular exercise that one can get on and stay with takes around 3 hours per week (Jonas, 1995, Tables 6.4, 6.5). For most weeks one half or more of the total training time is spent on the weekends. That may make things easier. But those "there's nothing to it, you can easily find the time" or "it really doesn't take any time at all" messages that accompany some exercise program recommendations, like those "no willpower messages accompanying various weight-loss programs," are not to be believed.

Regular exercise to a level that will provide significant benefits both for feeling good now and for future risk factor reduction does take time, regularly. Most people *can* find the time. But there has to be a *plan*, one has to *want* to do it, and your patient has to *take control*. And for few people it is that easy, at least in the beginning.

Finally, it is very important for both you and your patient/client to know and recognize that for most people who are trying to become regular exercisers, the chief problem is the regular, not the exercise. That is, getting on a regular, scheduled workout program and staying with it, not any technical aspect of the sport or activity itself, is the hardest part for most people. That is why my approach to training focuses at the beginning on the regular, not the exercise, on building a workout schedule into one's weekly routine first, using ordinary walking as the entry-level activity. For most people, once they can find-the-time/make-the-time on a regular basis, the rest, choosing and doing a sport or sports, an athletic activity or activities, is just commentary.

AEROBIC AND NONAEROBIC EXERCISE

WHAT "AEROBIC EXERCISE" IS

The most important point of this section is that exercise need not be done aerobically to be healthful and helpful (Concept IV). In the 1960s Dr. Kenneth Cooper coined the modern sense of the word "aerobic" and popularized the term and concept of aerobic exercise. The primary energy source for aerobic exercise is oxygen in breathed-in air, thus the word "aerobic" ("of the air"). But the term means more than simply using oxygen to support the muscular activity involved, because that is the case for nonaerobic exercise as well. In aerobic exercise, the muscles are "taking up," that is, using, a *significantly increased amount* of oxygen over what they normally do.

Exercising aerobically on a regular basis leads to improvement in two kinds of fitness: musculoskeletal and cardiovascular. *Musculoskeletal* fitness is the ability to do increased physical work over time using one or more major muscle groups. *Cardiovascular* fitness is the increased ability of the heart to beat faster and pump more blood with each beat, within the limits of healthy functioning, over time.

*Non*aerobic exercise is any physical activity above that of the normal resting state involving one or more major muscle groups that is sustained, but not so intense as to cause a significant increase in muscle oxygen uptake.* Like aerobic exercise, nonaerobic exercise can lead to an improvement in musculoskeletal fitness, although when done for the same amount of time obviously not as much, either in degree or potential endurance.

It was formerly thought that only aerobic exercise benefits the health of the heart over the long run. However, recent studies (Pratt, 1999) by Steven Blair and colleagues at the Cooper Institute in Dallas, Texas (Dunn, 1999) and Andersen et al. (1999) have demonstrated that regular "lifestyle exercise" (see below), can improve cardiovascular fitness and may reduce risk or coronary artery disease as well.

How One Knows If One Is Exercising Aerobically

Heart rate is a simple measure of the extent to which any exercise is aerobic. It is now generally considered that if one's heart rate reaches a level of 60% of the figure 220 minus your age (.6[220 − age]), one is exercising aerobically According to Wier and Jackson, this often-used formula only roughly approximates the true degree of increased oxygen uptake, however, (American Running Fitness Association, 1993), and is more accurate for beginning regular exercisers than experienced ones.

In any case, for the nonracing regular exerciser, qualitative measures of exercise intensity are perhaps even more useful than heart-rate monitoring. If one is breathing reasonably hard, or sweating while working out in mild to cold temperatures, it can be assumed that one is exercising aerobically. Most regular exercisers do not routinely take their pulse during a workout, relying rather on such subjective measures to know when they are "in the zone." At the top end, however, monitoring the pulse is a good idea. This is to make sure for safety's sake that one is not exercising at such an intensity

---

* *Non*aerobic exercise is different from *an*aerobic exercise. The latter does not use as its energy source breathed-in oxygen, but rather chemical energy stores already inside the muscles themselves. Anaerobic exercise, such as that done by sprinters, can be done very fast, but not for very long. Both aerobic and nonaerobic exercise can be done for very long periods of time. In the case of nonaerobic exercise, it is not simply done as fast as the aerobic variety.

that the heart rate goes above 85% of the theoretical maximum heart rate (once again, 220 – age), something to be avoided.

THE RELATIVE BENEFITS OF AEROBIC AND NON-AEROBIC EXERCISE

Most of the evidence to date shows that for exercise to be beneficial in terms of reducing long-term risk for coronary artery disease it must be aerobic (United States Department of Health and Human Services, 1996), although as noted above that picture may be changing (Pratt, 1999). However, even at a modest level of 1 to 2 hours per week of nonaerobic intensity, regular exercise is likely to be beneficial in reducing the risk of death from all causes (Blair et al., 1992; Rubin, 1999). And regular, even nonaerobic, exercise is definitely helpful for weight loss.

It is in fact becoming apparent that within the group of types of health-beneficial exercise, the major distinction is between planned, leisure-time, sport/activity-based regular exercise (aerobic or nonaerobic), and the "lifestyle" version (see below). There is no evidence to date that "lifestyle" exercise can confer the nonphysiological benefits of regular leisure-time exercise to the degree the latter can: feeling better, feeling better about yourself, getting the "postexercise" glow. And, of course, it is these benefits, not future risk-factor reduction, that keep most regular exercisers exercising regularly.

DO ALL REGULAR EXERCISERS EVENTUALLY DO IT AEROBICALLY?

No. It's possible that one may never become an aerobic exerciser, just an exerciser (Concept IV, again). Many people who have engaged in leisure-time scheduled regular exercise for years do it aerobically only on an intermittent basis, if at all. But they enjoy regular exercise anyway and still reap many of its here-and-now benefits. Most important for your patients/clients contemplating becoming regular exercisers is that whatever exercise pattern they settle on works for them.

The "Lifestyle" approach to exercise is incorporating extra exertion into one's daily pattern of living rather than blocking out time on a regular basis to do a sport or sport-related activity. Such exertion includes activities like using the stairs instead of the elevator, parking at the far end of the parking lot and walking the rest of the way to the office, getting off public transport a stop or two in advance of the usual one and walking the rest of the way, gardening, doing one's own housework, jogging in place for brief periods.

However, this is not magic. The activities must be done, to gain health benefits they must be done virtually every day (for about 30 minutes), and some time record must be kept. For some people, this may be the way to go to becoming a regular exerciser. But for many others, it will likely be easier over the long run to get on a program of vigorous leisure-time exercise employing a sport or sport-related activity, done regularly three to five times per week.

ROADBLOCKS THAT MAY BE ENCOUNTERED, AND HOW TO OVERCOME THEM

There are a series of roadblocks that may be encountered on the road to becoming a regular exerciser. If this happens, it is important to let your clients/patients know that they are not having a unique experience. Most regular exercisers have encountered more than one of them, and the many people who are now regular exercisers have successfully dealt with them.

Mental discipline, an important element of willpower (see chapter 5) is an essential element in becoming a regular exerciser. Two kinds of mental discipline are required. First, there is the mental discipline to start on something new, something that is challenging, and then stick with it, a subject we have spent much time on at various points throughout this book. At the same time, also needed is the mental discipline that athletes refer to as the ability to "stay within yourself." That is not overdoing it and trying to achieve something that is completely unrealistic, at least at the beginning.

SUPPOSE YOUR CLIENT SAYS, "I JUST DON'T LIKE THIS"

First, hone in on just what it is he/she doesn't like. Is it the regular? They should give themselves a fair shot at overcoming that hurdle. Perhaps they didn't spend enough time at the beginning "on the regular" (as discussed above) and got to the exercise part of the enterprise too soon. Perhaps they did get the regular down correctly, but then tried to do too much too soon when they got onto the exercise part, such as trying to go too long too early. You might try to refocus them on the "gradual change leads to permanent changes" approach. Finally, if it is the particular sport or activity with which they have started that they don't like, make them aware of the broad range that is available (Jonas, 1995, chapter 5).

SUPPOSE YOUR CLIENT SAYS, "IT HURTS"

Try first to figure out with them just what hurts. Is there an injury? As contrasted with the simple pain of muscle use and exertion, injury is often indicated by a good deal of pain in one area that doesn't go away, possibly accompanied by redness, swelling, and limitation of motion. If that is what your client is experiencing, he/she should stop working out and consult an appropriate health professional (who might turn out to be you, of course).

On the other hand, the pain may be the result only of exertion after long disuse and accompanying stiffness. Taking it easier and getting into it more slowly and gradually is the way to deal with this problem. A stretching program can be of great help (Jonas, 1995, pp. 120–125). In any case, at the beginning, it is far better to underdo it than to overdo it.

Pain may also be related to a problem with equipment, particularly shoes. A pair of shoes that doesn't fit can cause all sorts of problems, from shin splints to heel and toe blisters. Obviously, it is not desirable to go out first thing and spend a lot of money for a good pair of walking, running, or aerobics shoes if one is not really sure one is going to stick with it. But if they have nothing else around the house other than an old pair of sneakers (good for nothing other than increasing injury risk), they may have to do just that. Bad shoes that lead to pain and injury, which in turn lead to quitting, create a self-fulfilling prophecy.

Suppose Your Client Says, "I Don't Like Getting up Earlier in the Morning"

Regular exercisers have that experience all the time. Your client simply needs to know that the program will work, to have the mental discipline not to turn over in bed, snuggling under the covers for another 15 minutes, but to sit up, swing their legs over the side of the bed, splash some cold water on their face (or do whatever bathroom routine works for them), put on their stuff, and get out there. Again, the mental discipline—willpower—can be best reinforced by revisiting the assessment and goal setting process (Concept X).

Also, while it is not highly recommended, when starting out the majority of the minutes can be done on the weekends. And your client can stay with that arrangement until he/she is ready to increase the number of during-the-week workouts. Second, if working out in the morning is not attractive, one can consider going out before dinner or a bit after it.

Suppose Your Patient Simply Says, "This Is Just Not Working"

First, consider precisely what is meant by the term "not working." Does it mean not getting to look like Arnold or Cher within a month? Does it mean that the ultimate weight loss goal has not been reached in 2 months? Does it perhaps even mean only: "I don't understand it. I've been doing this stuff for 3 whole months [after a lifetime of living a sedentary lifestyle] and I'm not in tip-top shape yet." Does it thus really mean that immediate gratification is the true desire and it has not been achieved?

There is no easy way to deal with this one. The material on assessment, motivation, goal setting, success, and the natural history of health can be reviewed, reflecting of course on Concepts III, V, and X. And, remember that when starting from scratch, using the recommended one-step-at-a-time approach, if your client is like most people, he or she will not feel that they are "getting into shape" for at least 4 months, in many cases 6. These things just take time. Patience is important, for both your client/patient and for you.

MEASURING "SUCCESS" IN REGULAR EXERCISE

This is a subject that we have dwelt on at some length at various points throughout this book. That is because understanding it is so critical to achieving success in lifestyle/behavior change. First of all, the Concept that health has a natural history tells us that success in becoming a regular exerciser will not necessarily be the outcome of one's efforts at *any* given point in one's life, but only at *certain* ones. Those occur when one has mobilized one's motivation, has made the time, there is a physical place to exercise that is convenient, safe, and affordable, makes it fun, and so forth.

The essence of Concept V, discussed in chapter 4, is that a person's concept of "success" should be facilitating, not inhibiting. Thus to be helpful, in those behavior changes in which success is relative, like becoming a regular exerciser, success *must* be defined in terms relevant to the individual, to their present lifestyle, to what might *reasonably* be achieved, for themselves, not for anyone else. For example, if one is naturally slow afoot but decides to take up running, success should not be defined in terms of absolute speed, such as, "I will consider myself successful when I can run a mile in 8 minutes." Success in this case might be better defined in terms of endurance, such as, "As my first objective, I want to be able to run for 20 minutes without stopping, at a comfortable pace."

Once that objective is achieved, another can be set. It may be that *this* year your client's limit is to be able to handle the Stairmaster for 20 minutes without stopping, at a pace that gets his or her heart rate up to 50% of the "theoretic maximum" heart rate three times a week. Then *next* year the goal *can* be to get up to four 30-minute sessions per week at 60% of the theoretic maximum heart rate. Then, maybe 2 years down the road, as part of a multisport program, five times a week, he/she is going for 60 minutes or more at 70% of theoretic maximum heart rate and feeling just fine when the workout is over.

Do some people move along a continuum like this at a faster pace? Yes, they do. And that's fine, as long as they don't do it *too* quickly, get stressed-out, and quit. Staying in balance (Concept VII) is key to staying with it.

As far as endurance is concerned, after some reasonable stretch of training, say 3 to 4 months, most people will find that they can go quite a bit farther/longer in their chosen activity than they could have conceived of going before they got started. Often that is just a result of training itself. On the other hand, going fast is the product of training *plus* natural ability. Simply because of the way the human body is put together, many people simply will not be able to go very fast no matter how hard they try and how hard they train. To avoid frustration, injury, and quitting, it is important to recognize that fact.

To be able to recognize and accept one's limitations is a critical element in achieving success in athletics on one's own terms. Speed, strength, muscular bulk, flexibility, and gracefulness are in part achieved through training and practice. But as noted above in this chapter they are formed, too, in significant part by genetic make-up. Exactly what proportion of each achievement is determined by genetic endowment and what proportion by personal effort to build on it is not as yet known. But each of us does have genetically imposed limitations on what we can ultimately do with our bodies. It is very helpful, indeed sometimes liberating, to recognize them, at least in qualitative terms.

Whatever the relative weights are of endowment and enhancement in determining success, as noted above very few people have the genetic potential for developing the body of a world-class body builder (even if they were to use steroids), and very few have the potential of looking like a glamorous movie star (even with the assistance of plastic surgery). Nor do many people have it physically within themselves to run a marathon in under 3 hours. At the same time, many people have athletic potential, say for distance rather than speed, of which they were completely unaware. Thus, by engaging in endowment-enhancing activities, many can find within themselves the capability of doing things they never previously thought possible.

ACHIEVING BALANCE

As noted above, for most regular exercisers achieving balance (Concept VII) is a very important factor in staying with it. Some of your patients or clients may at some time have to work very hard mentally not to simply give it all up. Almost everyone who has worked through the process to become a regular exerciser still gets stale from time to time, still wakes up one morning wondering "why am I doing this?" and on occasion thinks "couldn't I be doing something better with my time?"

When that happens, it's time to reevaluate. These thoughts are often the result of some kind of *imbalance* creeping into the activity. Is the person trying too hard? Have they set unrealistic goals? Are they hurting or getting injured? In other words, are they becoming *unbalanced* in what they are doing? Is it time perhaps to change sports or add a new one (that is getting into what is called "cross-training")?

The best way to avoid this is to suggest, one (reassessment and revisiting their initial assessment), that they think back to what their body and mind were like before they became a regular exerciser (do they really want to be in that place again?), and two (revisiting goal setting), that they make some changes in their program and sports. Even if everything is going great, it is a good idea to reevaluate periodically. What they really want to be sure of is: "Have I achieved success in this endeavor and am I happy with where I am?" In other words, have they achieved balance in their own exercise regimen?

Regular exercise should lead to improved health and fitness, and to feeling good. It should not lead to injury, anxiety, frustration, anger, isolation, and stress. Regular exercise should help to manage life's stresses better. It should not be a *cause* of stress. Dealing with exercise as a stress*or* is much the same as handling it as a cause of over-use injury: cut down on the amount and the intensity of training. Just as balance is the key to health, so too is it the key to healthy exercise.

If a person has it within themselves to become a good athlete (whether "good" is defined by speed or by endurance, by winning or by simply participating) as well as a regular exerciser, that athletic ability will come out in good time. And then more time will be found for sport. All in good time. You can be sure of that.

ON TAKING A BREAK FROM TIME TO TIME

Overdoing it either when starting out or when well underway is much worse than cutting down from time to time. Sometimes we get stale. Once one becomes fit, to lose all conditioning would take not working out at all for a 3- to 5-month period (American College of Sports Medicine, 1992, p. 99). At the same time, an important part of mental discipline for the regular exerciser is to be able to recognize when a break is needed and when it's simply necessary to push. Trial and error is the only way to develop this skill.

ON KNOWING WHEN TO STOP

Suppose that your client has given regular exercise a reasonable and legitimate try. But he or she finds that it just isn't fun. He can't get on a regular schedule. She can't find an enjoyable sport or activity. In addition, one finds that one is not experiencing the advertised benefits, or that whatever reward derived just does not justify the effort. If this is the case, the best thing to do is stop, at least for the present. And you should give your patient permission to do so. No guilt and no guilt-trips.

In theory, regular exercise, aerobic or nonaerobic, is good for almost everyone. But maybe it just isn't in the cards for a given client at a given time. Perhaps that inner motivation isn't really there yet. Maybe 6 to 12 months from now your client will feel differently. But perhaps she never will. That's okay. Maybe, for example, the time *really* just isn't available in a very busy schedule. Not being a regular exerciser doesn't make one a bad person. There are many good people who are not regular exercisers.

If one just doesn't feel like doing it or is not getting very much out of it, then they should stop. If in this state they try to continue, they will likely become angry and frustrated and will certainly raise their risk of injury. Maybe your patient or client will be able to get back to it at some time in the future. Maybe they never will. But at least the client will have the knowledge that he or she did try.

USING THE TEN CONCEPTS

Let us conclude this chapter with a brief review of how all of the Ten Concepts, not just the ones specifically discussed in the text, have applicability to a discussion of regular exercise with your patients and clients.

Regular exercise is important to maintaining and improving the state of being that is health (Concept I). It is also a central to that process of being known as wellness. However, because health status is determined by a broad range of factors (and there is a variety of engines to help move one along the wellness pathway), if one cannot exercise regularly for a variety of reasons, or simply does not want to, that does not mean that on balance one cannot be both healthy and well (Concept II).

That health has a natural history tells us that individuals can come to regular exercise at virtually any stage of life, and just because one is not ready or capable of starting at time A, that does not mean that they will not get going at time B or C (Concept III). Not only are a wide array of interventions central to the wellness process, but within one group, in this case "regular exercise," there are also many variants (Concept IV).

Certainly success is a relative term in regular exercise (Concept V). Regular exercise reduces the risks for a wide variety of negative health conditions; but there is certainly no certainty of outcome (Concept VI) (except that in most cases practitioners of vigorous regular exercise do feel better, look better, and feel better about themselves). As we have seen, achieving balance is essential to success is regular exercise (Concept VII).

The road to becoming a regular exerciser clearly follows the common Stages of Change pathway to success for most personal behavior change efforts (Concept VIII). The Concept (IX) that motivation is a process, not a thing, is clearly illustrated by the process of becoming a regular exerciser. And finally (Concept X), assessment, goal setting, and mobilizing motivation are central to the task of becoming a regular exerciser.

REFERENCES

ACSM: American College of Sports Medicine. (1992). *ACSM fitness book.* Champaign, IL: Human Kinetics/Leisure Press.

American College of Sports Medicine. (1999). *ACSM guidelines.* Dallas, TX: The Cooper Institute for Aerobics Research.

American Running and Fitness Association. (1993). Exercise intensity: Misleading measurements. *Running and FitNews, 11,* 1.

Andersen, R. E., et al. (1999). Effects of lifestyle activity vs. structured aerobic exercise in obese women. *Journal of the American Medical Association, 281,* 335–340.

Blair, S. N., Kohl, H. W., Gordon, N. F., & Paffenbarges, R. S., Jr. (1992). How much physical activity is good for health? *Annual Review of Public Health, 13,* 99–126.

Cooper, K. (1985). *Running without fear.* New York: M. Evans and Co.

Cooper, K., quoted in Hanc, J. (1994, October 8). Too much pain, maybe no gain, *Newsday,* B7.

Dunn, A. L. (1999). Comparison of lifestyle and structure interventions to increase physical activity and cardiorespiratory fitness. *Journal of the American Medical Association, 281,* 327–334.

Jonas, S. (1995). *Regular exercise: A handbook for clinical practice.* New York: Springer Publishing.

Pratt, M. (1999). Benefits of lifestyle activity vs. structured exercise. *Journal of the American Medical Association, 281,* 375–376.

Rubin, A. (1999). Daily accumulated exercise improves adult fitness. *The Physician and Sports Medicine, 27,* 27.

US Department of Health and Human Services. (1996). *Physical activity and health: A report of the surgeon general.* Atlanta, GA: Centers for Disease Control and Prevention.

United States Preventive Services Task Force. (1996). *Guide to clinical preventive services: Report of the US preventive services task force* (2nd ed.) Baltimore, MD: Williams and Wilkins.

Chapter 8

INCORPORATING HEALTH PROMOTION/DISEASE PREVENTION INTO YOUR PRACTICE: A PROCESS OF PERSONAL CHANGE

I. INTRODUCTION

OVERVIEW

For many health care practitioners trained in traditional, disease-oriented Western medicine, incorporating both health promotion/disease prevention (HP/DP) functions and an attention to wellness into their practices constitutes a major behavior change. It is not a simple one, and should not be undertaken lightly. Interestingly enough, the process a practitioner needs to go through to effect this change in his or her pattern of work is similar to that which a patient/client making a personal HP/DP lifestyle/behavior change goes through. The parallels between the two processes are in fact fascinating.

In this chapter, we shall discuss briefly the process of adding a HP/DP and wellness focus to one's mode of professional practice.

First, we shall consider the application to the professional change process of those of the Ten Central Concepts of Health Promotion/Disease Prevention that are relevant to that process. Then, bearing that application in mind, we shall review a series of questions that will help us work through the professional change process for ourselves.

WHO

Recall that throughout this book we have been looking at that central body of knowledge, skills, and attitudes in supporting personal HP/DP-oriented practice that is useful for all health care practitioners engaged in it. Although there are certainly variations in the complexity of that central body that vary with one's level of responsibility, the essence of the change process each type of practitioner wishing to incorporate HP/DP functions into his/her work needs to experience is much the same. This is so whether the practitioner is a physician (MD/DO), a dentist, a dental hygienist, a chiropractor, a nurse or nurse practitioner, a physicians' assistant or associate, a health educator, a social worker, a psychologist, a physical or occupational therapist, a nutritionist, an exercise physiologist, a certified addiction counsellor, or a member of any other health profession or health-related occupation that deals with HP/DP in the care of patients or clients.

WHAT

As noted especially in chapter five, for most of the personal HP/DP interventions there is a common set of functions that, to a greater or lesser extent depending upon the health care provider's specific role, needs to be undertaken. To review that briefly, in patient/client evaluation there are the HP/DP-oriented history, any relevant physical examination, and laboratory and machine-based testing as indicated. The results of this evaluation will enable the creation of a HP/DP and wellness-related problem list and an estimate of the patient/client's behavior change Stage and capability.

The available primary personal HP/DP interventions include: direct medical service, such as planned maintenance of immune status, treatment of hypertension, family planning/prenatal care/infant and child care; patient/client education/counselling on an individual or group basis, both for risk factor modification and for developing a wellness lifestyle; and provision of or referral to community-based HP/DP facilities and programs of various kinds (e.g., gyms, smoking cessation, weight loss programs).

As we have said on numerous occasions in this book (but it is a point well worth repeating), it is vitally important to be aware of, and make the patient/client aware of, the commonalities behind the ways in which many negative health habits can be dealt with: The process that begins with assessment, continues with goal setting and mobilizing motivation, and then (hopefully) on to changing behavior, and is central to managing all health-related problems that can be dealt with using personal behavior change.

WHERE

Settings for the provision of HP/DP services include: private health care offices (general and dedicated HP/DP practices, e.g., behavioral medicine centers); health care institutions (hospitals, HMOs [both group and office-based], long-term care facilities); worksites (both dedicated and non-dedicated facilities/services); community-based services (can be for-profit/not-for-profit; single-purpose/multipurpose; primary function/one of many functions); educational institutions (primary and secondary-schools; technical schools; universities, at the undergraduate and graduate levels); in the home and on the media, both print and electronic.

ROLE-MODELING

Does a practitioner need to be a picture of health himself or herself in order to engage in a health-oriented practice? The answer is: No, but it helps. It helps from a practical standpoint. The practitioner can then speak with personal as well as professional experience about the subject at hand, whether it be something as challenging as becoming a regular exerciser or as relatively simple as learning to fasten your seatbelt every time you get in the car. It also helps from the "showing-the-flag" standpoint. But, just as it is very important not to use guilt as a motivator in dealing with clients and patients, so it is very important not to use guilt when dealing with oneself on one's professional role. It works in neither context. Role modeling for HP/DP by health care practitioners is a functional matter, not a moral one.

Given that role-modeling is useful in a HP/DP and wellness-oriented practice, does that mean that the overweight professional can never talk with an overweight patient about weight loss? By all means, no. If, for example, the professional has attempted to lose weight without success, but engages in other health-promoting personal behaviors, he/she has two special perspectives to offer patients and clients.

One is how difficult it is to lose weight, so that if the patient/client is successful they can look upon the achievement as something really special. The other is that personal health is the product of a spectrum of behaviors and other health-related factors (Concept II), and thus (morbid obesity excluded) it is quite possible to be overweight and healthy at the same time.

II. APPLYING SELECTED CONCEPTS TO THE PRACTITIONER'S CHANGE PROCESS

Reviewing the substantive Concepts, we find that numbers I, III, V, and VII apply to the process that the practitioner adding the HP/DP and wellness functions to their armamentarium experiences.

I. HEALTH IS A STATE OF BEING; WELLNESS IS A PROCESS OF BEING

The "health" of your HP/DP-oriented practice is its "state of being" in relation to the degree of focus placed upon HP/DP and wellness at any given time. Like personal health, that focus can be measured and evaluated. The "wellness" of your HP/DP-oriented practice is a characterization of the professional development process in that arena you are engaged in over time. Paralleling the process of personal wellness, what can be called "professional wellness" is a process of continuing growth, broadening horizons, and deepening understanding of HP/DP and how its incorporation into virtually any kind of health care practice helps our patients and clients. Like personal wellness, it is a process that never ends.

III. Health has A Natural History

Also ongoing is the change process for your practice. Just as a patient/client may be ready now to make a major behavior change, or may not be ready for two years, so may you be ready now, or not be ready for two years. And in each case, that's OK. For any of us, changing the way we engage in our particular health-related practice is something that takes time, over time. There is no one timetable that applies to everyone. If you want to get started on making this major change in how you practice, like the patient/client making a personal lifestyle/behavior change you will know when you are ready to do so. Then you will proceed, at your own pace.

V. Success in Certain Behavior Change
Endeavors Is Relative

Recall that for personal HP/DP there are certain absolutes: e.g., no nicotine/tobacco use, no abuse of the other recreational mood-altering drugs. In a HP/DP-oriented practice, obviously whatever it is that we do should be of high technical quality. But in terms of the content of the HP/DP and wellness-oriented practice, just as there are no absolute standards by which to measure "success" for any one patient engaging in, say, weight loss or regular exercise, so are there no absolute standards for measuring success in changing one's practice.

That is, there are no fixed requirements that a health-oriented practice must, for example, include exercise promotion or weight management, or any other specific element. You will choose those with which you are comfortable and which you think will work for your clients/patients. And you can always add others as you go along, should you choose to do so.

For the typical disease-oriented practitioner, any well-done HP/DP practice-component represents an advance over his/her previous approach to care delivery. "Success" in changing your practice orientation thus needs to be characterized in terms of what *you* can reasonably be expected to be able to accomplish in *your* practice, over time, given its realities.

VII. Achieving Balance Is the Essence of Healthy Living and Wellness

Just as the healthy and well person will strive for balance in their life and in their approach to health and wellness, so should the HP/DP-oriented practitioner strive for balance in their practice. For example, as primarily disease-oriented practitioners like physicians and dentists come to focus more on health, they should be careful not to go overboard in that regard, and end up throwing the baby out with the bathwater. Too much "health," at the expense of expected and necessary attention to disease in their patient population will do patients no more good than does the current overemphasis on disease care in many medical practices.

Turning now to the process Concepts, we find that all three apply to the practice-change endeavor.

VIII. There Is A Common Pathway to Success for Most Personal Behavior Change Efforts

So too is there one for the health care practitioner wishing to change how they do their work. Each of us goes through a professional version of the Stages of Change progression. At the beginning of your own change process, just as any patient/client does, you need to figure out where you are in it. If you are thinking about making a change, you are obviously past Pre-Contemplation. But are you now in Contemplation, or Preparation, or on the verge of Action? Given that there is a common change process, knowing where you are on the Stage of Change continuum will help you to achieve success, as you define it for yourself.

IX. MOTIVATION IS A PROCESS, NOT A THING

Motivation is just as central to professional behavior change as it is to personal behavior change—and it is of the same nature. To review, it is the process that links a thought, e.g., "I would like to start incorporating stress management assistance into my practice," with the action of actually doing so. You can no more make HP/DP-oriented changes in your practice without mobilizing your motivation to do so than a patient or client of yours can stop smoking without mobilizing his or her motivation to do that. And just as patient change does, so does professional change take conviction, understanding, dedication, and—yes—willpower.

X. ASSESSMENT, GOAL SETTING, AND MOBILIZING MOTIVATION ARE THE CENTRAL TASKS IN PERSONAL BEHAVIOR CHANGE

And finally, these three tasks of Concept X are as central to a practitioner's own behavior change process as they are to personal HP/DP behavior change. First, assessment. For example, in your practice, what is the list of patient/client needs for HP/DP interventions and guidance on the wellness road? Which of them are you meeting? Which ones not? Of the list of unmet patient needs that you have assembled, which do you think you might be able to meet now, in six months, in one year, in five years?

Having done that review, you will then go on to set goals for yourself, designed to meet the identified unmet needs. And it is just as important for you to spend considerable time doing that as it is for the patients in the Preparation Stage of personal behavior change to spend considerable time on goal setting. Also, as noted, just as we use "reasonableness" in goal setting for patients, your practice goals must be ones that you, not some other practitioner, can reasonably expect to achieve in a reasonable period of time.

In doing this you have to be sure to take into account: your own level of interest and knowledge; the available time and space; the adequacy of supporting staff, if required; and any payment/financing considerations that must be dealt with. Finally, to make the planned practice changes, you will mobilize your motivation in just the same way the client/patient making a personal lifestyle/ behavior change does.

III. FORMULATING QUESTIONS

To help you go through the process of professional behavior change, of developing and implementing a plan for incorporating health promotion/disease prevention and the wellness philosophy into your clinical practice at a level that is useful for your patients/clients and comfortable for you, here is a series of questions for you to ask and answer for yourself (see also Westberg and Jason, 1996, pp. 150–152).

- Is HP/DP important in my practice, and why? For which patients/clients?
- For any endeavor in this area, what are the goals I want to achieve, for my patients/clients, for myself, for the practice?
- If I think that there is some new stuff to learn here, how much time do I want to invest in doing so, if any? And if not I, then who?
- Who should do the counselling? I? Members of my staff? Somebody new whom I might bring in part-time, like (for a physician) a health educator or a nutritionist with a broad interest in HP/DP?
- Whoever does it, how is this function going to be paid for? Do I charge patients for this service? If so, how?
- Do I want to try patient groups for certain interventions, like promoting regular exercise or smoking cessation? What about using community resources?
- How much time am I willing to invest in developing a HP/DP component in my practice?
- Is role modeling important? If so, by whom? Do I want to invest my personal time in this?
- In terms of the specifics, how should I go about learning them, incorporating them into my own knowledge, thinking, and pattern of practice?

If you decide to undertake the journey towards a health-oriented practice, it will likely be one upon which you will be very happy to have embarked. And for that journey, I wish you *bon voyage*!

REFERENCES

Westberg, J., & Jason, H. (1996). Influencing health behavior: The process. In S. H. Woolf, S. Jonas, & R. Lawrence (Eds.), *Health promotion and disease prevention in clinical practice* (pp. 145–162). Baltimore, MD: Williams and Wilkins.

RESOURCES

I. BOOKS ON HEALTH PROMOTION AND DISEASE PREVENTION, GENERAL

Agency for Health Care Policy and Research. (1998). *Clinician's Handbook of Preventive Services*. Washington, DC: US Dept. of Health and Human Services, Office of Public Health and Science, 1998.

Berkman, L. F., & Breslow, L. (1983). *Health and ways of living: The Alameda County study*. New York: Oxford University Press.

Bouchard, C., Shepard, R. J., & Stephens, T., (Eds.). (1988). *Physical activity, fitness, and health: International proceedings and consensus statement*. Champaign, IL: Human Kinetics Publishers.

Downie, R. S., Tannahill, C., & Tannahill, A. (1996). *Health promotion: Models and values*. Oxford, England: Oxford University Press.

Gorin, S. S., & Arnold, J. (1998). *Health Promotion Handbook*. St. Louis, MO: Mosby.

Hagen, P. T. (1997). *Mayo HealthQuest: Guide to self-care*. Rochester, MN: Mayo Foundation for Medical Education and Research.

Kassberg, M., & Jonas, S. (1999). *Help your man get healthy: An essential guide for every caring woman*. New York: Whole Care/Avon Books.

United States Preventive Services Task Force (1996). *Guide to clinical preventive services: Report of the US preventive services task force* (2nd ed.). Baltimore, MD: Williams and Wilkins.

Woolf, S. H., Jonas, S., & Lawrence, R., (Eds.). (1996). *Health promotion and disease prevention in clinical practice*. Baltimore, MD: Williams and Wilkins.

World Health Organization (1958). *The World Health Organization: A report on the first ten years*. Geneva, Switzerland.

II. BOOKS ON HEALTH PROMOTION, SUBJECT-SPECIFIC

ACSM: American College of Sports Medicine (1998). *ACSM fitness book* (2nd ed.). Champaign, IL: Human Kinetics.

ACSM: American College of Sports Medicine (1999). *ACSM guidelines*. Dallas, TX: The Cooper Institute for Aerobics Research.

American Heart Association (1997). *Fitting in fitness*. New York: Times Books.

Clark, N. (1997). *Nancy Clark's Sports Nutrition Guidebook*. Champaign, IL: Human Kinetics.

Cooper, K. (1982). *The aerobics program for total wellbeing*. New York: Bantam Books.

Jonas, S. (1993). *Take control of your weight*. Yonkers, NY: Consumers Reports Books.

Jonas, S. (1995). *Regular exercise: A handbook for clinical practice*. New York: Springer Publishing. (An abridged version for patients/ clients, *A Guidebook for the Regular Exerciser* is also available.)

Jonas, S., & Konner, L. (1997). *Just the weigh you are: How to be fit and healthy, whatever your size*. Boston, MA: Chapters Publishing/ Houghton Mifflin.

Laliberte, R., George, S.C., and the Editors of Men's Health Books. (1997). *The men's health guide to peak conditioning*. Emmaus, PA: Rodale Press.

Long, B., et al., (1992). *Project PACE: Physician-based assessment and counseling for exercise*. Atlanta, GA: Centers for Disease Control and Prevention.

United States Department of Health and Human Services. (1996). *Physical activity and health: A report of the surgeon general*. Atlanta, GA: Centers for Disease Control and Prevention.

United States Department of Health and Human Services, Centers for Disease Control and Prevention. (1999). *Promoting physical activity: A guide for community action*. Champaign, IL: Human Kinetics Press.

III. BOOKS ON WELLNESS

Ardell, D. B. (1984). *The History and Future of Wellness*. Pleasant Hill, CA: Diablo Press.

Ardell, D. B. (1986). *High level wellness: An alternative to doctors, drugs, and disease*. Berkeley, CA: Ten Speed Press.

Ardell, D. B. (1996). *The Book of Wellness: A Secular Approach to Spirit, Meaning & Purpose*. Amherst, NY: Prometheus Books.

Clark, C. C. (1996). *Wellness Practitioner: Concepts, Research and Strategies*. New York: Springer Publishing.

Dunn, H. L. (1961, 1977). *High-Level Wellness*. Thorofare, NJ: Charles B. Slack.

Kass-Annese, B. (1997). *A total wellness program for women over 30: Comprehensive manual with medical guidelines for health care professionals*. New York: Springer Publishing.

Ryan, R. S., & Travis, J. W. (1991). *Wellness: Small changes you can use to make a big difference*. Berkeley, CA: Ten Speed Press.

IV. BOOKS ON COMPLEMENTARY/ ALTERNATIVE MEDICINE

Clark, C. C. (Ed.). (1999). *Encyclopedia of complementary health practice*. New York: Springer Publishing.

Clark, C. C. (2000). *Integrating complementary health procedures into practice*. New York: Springer Publishing.

Gordon, R. J., Nienstedt, B. C., Gesler, W. M. (1998). *Alternative therapies: Exploring options in health care*. New York: Springer Publishing.

Snyder, M., & Lindquist, R. (1998). *Complementary/alternative therapies in nursing* (3rd ed.). New York: Springer Publishing.

V. THE FEDERAL "HEALTHY PEOPLE" INITIATIVE

United States Department of Health, Education, and Welfare. (1979). *Healthy people: The surgeon general's report on health promotion and disease prevention*. Washington, DC: Author. (Pub. No. 79–55071).

United States Department of Health and Human Services (1991). *Healthy people 2000: National health promotion and disease prevention objectives*. Washington, DC: US Public Health Service. (DHHS Pub. No. [PHS] 91-50213).

United States Department of Health and Human Services. (1995). *Healthy people 2000: Mid-course review and 1995 revisions.* Washington, DC: U.S. Public Health Service.

United States Department of Health and Human Services. (1998). *Health, United States, 1998, with socioeconomic status and health chartbook.* Hyattsville, MD: National Center for Health Statistics. (DHHS Pub. No. (PHS) 98-1232; this publication is issued periodically.)

United States Department of Health and Human Services. (1998, Sept. 15) *Healthy people 2010 objectives: Draft for public comment.* Washington, DC: Office of Public Health and Science.

United States Department of Health and Human Services. (1999, June). *Healthy people 2000 review 1998–99.* Hyattsville, MD: Centers for Disease Control and Prevention. (DHHS Pub. No. (PHS) 99-1256).

VI. JOURNALS

ACSM's Health and Fitness Journal
UNLV College of Health Sciences
PO Box 453034
Las Vegas, NV 89154-3034

Alternative Health Practitioner: The Journal of Complementary and Natural Care
Springer Publishing Company
536 Broadway
New York, NY 10012

American Journal of Health Promotion
1660 Cass Lake Road, Suite 104
Keego Harbor, MI 48320

American Medical Athletics Association Quarterly
4405 East-West Highway
Suite 405
Bethesda, MD 20814

American Journal of Preventive Medicine
San Diego State University
5500 Campanile Drive
San Diego, CA 92182-4710

American Journal of Public Health
    800 I St., NW
    Washington, D.C. 20001-3710

Healthy Weight Journal
    402 S. 14th Street
    Hettinger, ND 58639

Journal of Nutrition, Health, and Aging: An International Journal
    Springer Publishing Company
    536 Broadway
    New York, NY 10012

Morbidity and Mortality Weekly Report
    Centers for Disease Control and Prevention
    1600 Clifton Road, N.E.
    Atlanta, GA 30333

Preventive Medicine
    Academic Press
    525 B Street, Suite 1900
    San Diego, CA 92101-4495

The Physician and Sportsmedicine
    McGraw-Hill
    4530 W. 77th Street
    Minneapolis, MN 55435

VII. NEWSLETTERS

The Ardell Wellness Report
    Dr. Don Ardell
    345 Bayshore
    Tampa, FL 33606

The Art of Health Promotion
    c/o American Journal of Health Promotion (supra)

Health Promotion: Global Perspectives
  c/o American Journal of Health Promotion (supra)

Nutrition Action
  Center for Science in the Public Interest
  1875 Connecticut Avenue N.W., Suite 300
  Washington, D.C. 20009-5728

Running and FitNews
  4405 East-West Highway
  Suite 405
  Bethesda, MD 20814

University of California Berkeley Wellness Letter
  Health Letter Associates
  Box 412, Prince Street Station
  New York, NY 10012-0007

Weight Control Digest
  American Health Publishing Co.
  1110 S. Airport Circle, Suite 110
  Euless, TX 76040

Wellness Management
  National Wellness Association
  PO Box 827
  Stevens Point, WI 54481-0827

Worksite Wellness Works
  Health Insurance Association of America
  1850 K Street, N.W.
  Washington, D.C. 20006-2284

VIII. WEB SITES (examples; address may not be current)

"Ask the Wellness Expert," Dr. Donald Ardell
  www.yourhealth.com

Ball State University Institute for Wellness
  www.bsu.edu/wellness/

National Wellness Association
  www.wellnesswi.org/nwa/

National Wellness Institute
www.nationalwellness.org

State University of New York at Buffalo Living Well Center
www.student-health.buffalo.edu/lwc

University of Wisconsin at Stevens Point Wellness Center
www.wellness.uwsp.edu

IX. PROFESSIONAL ASSOCIATIONS

American College of Preventive Medicine
1660 L St., N.W., Suite 206
Washington, D.C. 20036–5603
(202) 466–2044

American Medical Athletics Association
4405 East-West Highway
Suite 405
Bethesda, MD 20814
(301) 913–9517

American Public Health Association
800 I St., NW
Washington, D.C. 20001–3710
(202) 777–APHA

Association of Teachers of Preventive Medicine
1660 L St., N.W., Suite 208
Washington, D.C. 20036–5603
Phone: (202) 463–0550
Fax: 463–0555

National Wellness Institute
1045 Clark St., Suite 210
PO Box 827
Stevens Point, WI 54481–0827
Phone: (715) 342–2969
Fax: (715) 342–2979

INDEX

Abandonment, of positive behavior, temporary, lapse as, 70
Action, in process of change, 69
Addictive drug, nicotine as, 17
Advertising
 of alcohol, 42
 of tobacco, 17
Aerobic exercise, 110–113
 defined, 110–111
AIDS, prevention of, 38
Air pollution, 36
Airbags, in automobile, 17
Alcohol, 31, 54
 advertising, 42
 driving drunk, 17
 use of by children, 42
Alcoholism, cost of, 38
Ambivalence
 in change process, 68
 dealing with, 82–83
American College of Preventive Medicine, name, address of, 137
American Medical Athletics Association, name, address of, 137
American Public Health Association, name, address of, 137
Antibiotics, introduction of, 34
Apollo, significance of, 11
Ardell Wellness Report, publication of, 20
Asklepios
 followers of, 11–12
 significance of, 12

Assessment, in behavior change, 75–76
Association of Teachers of Preventive Medicine, name, address of, 137
Automobile
 airbags in, 17
 collision, personal injury from, 17
 safe design, governmental requirements for, 18
 seat belts, increased use of, 35

Balance, 95–97
 disturbed, disease as, 11
 as goal, 62–64
 health as, 11–12
 with outside world, 13
Beauty ideal, thinness as, 54
Behavior
 change, 59–61, 94
  common pathway to success, 67
 patterns, effect on health, 17
 positive, abandonment, temporary, lapse as, 70
Bill of Rights, wellness and, 20
Cancer, 17, 61
 as cause of death, 31
Cardiovascular fitness, 110
Causes of death, by medical diagnosis, 31
Cervical screening, 28
Change, stages of, 67, 99, 102–103
Chemotherapy, positive effect of, 33
Children, use of tobacco, alcohol by, 42
Christianity, rise of, approach to health during, 12

139